PAIN
WITH
POISE

PAIN
WITH
POISE

A TRACTOR-TRAILER ACCIDENT,
A JOURNEY OF RESTORATION,
AND A LIFE FOREVER CHANGED

Ashley Swartzwelder

Copyright © 2024 by Ashley Swartzwelder

This book, or parts thereof, may not be
reproduced in any form without permission. All rights reserved.
Unauthorized duplication is a violation of applicable law.

Disclaimer: The author's opinions, comments, and criticisms expressed herein are based on his personal observations and his research and readings on the subject matter. The author's opinions, comments, and criticisms may not be universally applicable to all people in all circumstances. The information presented in this book is intended as general information for educational purposes only and should not be construed as medical advice or diagnosis of any kind or as a substitute for medical or psychological treatment. The information should be used in conjunction with the guidance and care of your physician. Do not rely upon any information to replace consultations or advice provided by qualified health professionals. The publisher and author disclaim liability for any negative or other medical or psychological outcomes that may occur as a result of acting on or not acting on anything set forth in this book. The information in this book is not to be used to provide advice or attempt a diagnosis for the author.

Photos on page 39 by Jennifer Walters.

For more information, go to the author's website at
www.ashleyswartzwelder.com.

Paperback ISBN: 978-1-63337-912-1
E-book ISBN: 978-1-63337-822-3

Printed in the United States of America
1 3 5 7 9 10 8 6 4 2

TO EDEN
May every dream be granted

TABLE OF CONTENTS

Preface..I

Part 1: The Accident and the Aftermath..........................1

Chapter 1: Perspectives..3
Chapter 2: The First Year of Physical Suffering................13
Chapter 3: Energy, Force, and Interconnectedness............19
Chapter 4: Taking Life for Granted................................39
Chapter 5: The Alchemy of my Body from Trauma...........43
Chapter 6: The Slap...63
Chapter 7: Sanity in an Insane World............................65
Chapter 8: Life and Relationships After Trauma...............69
Chapter 9: Healthcare Horrors......................................79
Chapter 10: Professionally Limited................................99
Chapter 11: Dating in the Trauma World.....................115
Chapter 12: The Evolving "I".....................................117
Chapter 13: The COVID-19 Pandemic.......................125
Chapter 14: Energy, Research, and Intellect..................135
Chapter 15: Diet and Nutrition..................................153
Chapter 16: The Transition..159
Chapter 17: Justice..163

Part 2: Rehabilitation in Detail............................167

Chapter 18: Visualization & Physical Rehabilitation........171
Chapter 19: The Mirage of Poise...............................187
Chapter 20: Breathing Rehabilitation.......................201
Chapter 21: Core Rehabilitation..............................211
Chapter 22: Neck Rehabilitation.............................241
Chapter 23: Weight Rehabilitation..........................269
Chapter 24: Lower Body Rehabilitation....................275
Chapter 25: Balance Rehabilitation.........................289
Chapter 26: Running Rehabilitation........................295
Chapter 27: Resources & The Science of the Accident......301

Acknowledgments...309
Bibliography..311
Endnotes..319
About the Author..329

We are but falsehood, duplicity and contradiction, using even to ourselves concealment and guile.
—*Blaise Pascal*[1]

PREFACE

In 2005, I stood facing the chalkboard and dropped my head in defeat. It was over.

I had failed my first-year chemistry oral exam at The Ohio State University. I couldn't answer the one and only question that the examining committee had asked. It happened to be regarding energy. My only answer was the basic energy equation. I had stood for 20 minutes being grilled about the same question. During those long minutes, I recalled one of the horror stories that floated around before oral exams. This one student had run out of her first-year oral exam because hers had been so horrible. I was not going to be that student. With my back to the examining team, I waited until I was dismissed, and I walked out.

After my miserable performance, I decided I would be a success in graduate school. In 2006, I defended my master's research and received an "impressive" from one of the professors on my examining committee. I began celebrating my approaching graduation. I had redeemed myself. To accomplish my master's degree, I had overcome many challenges throughout my life. A few began as a child. One challenge was a speech impediment. For that, I attended speech therapy. With time it resolved, but I still utilize cues to assist my speech to this day. I was also diagnosed with epilepsy in high school. Epilepsy didn't scare me, and not many people knew I had it. Even with this disease, I could live like everyone else. That made me really happy. I never considered myself to be different.

PAIN WITH POISE

After graduation, I accepted a job at Chemical Abstracts Service where I analyzed scientific information from intellectual properties and peer-reviewed journals from international publications. I developed an expertise in geology, analytical chemistry, nuclear engineering, and nuclear physics. These areas of science became my passion. My love for my job fueled my interest in public policy. While I enjoyed my work, I chose to resign in November 2016. I desired a career change, yet I couldn't decide what I wanted to do. I decided to call it a professional sabbatical to explore leadership.

During my 10-year tenure at Chemical Abstracts Service, I got married and divorced. My husband became a police officer and had become increasingly emotionally abusive. He was also having an online affair and who knows what else. I decided to give him two options: a dissolution or a separation to work on things. He chose a dissolution.

I remember sharing that I had gotten a divorce on social media. A total stranger reached out asking how to get a divorce themselves. I told them what to do. While I don't know what came of my advice, I immediately embraced this gift I called *voice*. I realized I had a duty to drop my comfortable life and become more transparent about taboo topics. There were people looking for a person who was willing to step outside of a comfort zone to discuss difficult topics. This gift became my responsibility. It became a journey into human and civil rights. I decided to transition into political activism.

Transitioning into political activism was an exciting journey. I approached issues like I always had—with an open-minded perspective. This allowed me to consider all possible reasons for behaviors. Open-minded thinkers, like world-renowned researchers, break the status quo. As a society, it benefited us to embrace each fleeting moment as an opportunity to learn, adjust, and enhance our own lives and society. However, while everyone else focused on "others," they forgot about the importance of themselves in the equation.

PREFACE

In 2017, I began developing a philosophy about *It's All About the "I."* I knew that every human was an intellectual being. Even though each human was born with different levels of intelligence, they had the ability to expose themselves to different people, cultures, and events. Being curious and flexible, yet grounded, with each interaction, provided a learning atmosphere if open to evolving. As a result, a well-rounded growth in all intelligences, also referred to as SECCI (social, emotional, cultural, and contextual intelligences), would be observed. This would provide universally guided, intuitive insight in all forms of human and non-human encounters.

My leadership sabbatical was progressing well. Then in May 2018, I was hit by a tractor-trailer, a cab tractor carrying a trailer loaded with 40 tons of freight. In one second, I became a new person. In my head, there was a monster. My face was a monster. The foreign body was a monster. My walk was a monster's walk. My speech was a monster's speech. My actions were a monster's actions. I was a monster, and monster was me. My monster now lived with me. Both of us faced the challenges of life together.

I had to face the challenge of developing, because I felt like Frankenstein's monster.[1] The semi-trailer truck had shredded me. The person I believed I was and portrayed myself to be was gone. I no longer recognized myself or my life. Instead I encountered the being that lived inside, hidden—the being all living were forever denied the ability to embrace. And for a reason, this person was a monster. As such, I learned to value the human life differently. My recovery was all about the "I." I quickly realized that to heal, I needed innovation in all areas to achieve my dreams. I was desperate to find a team that could get rid of monster as fast as possible. My monsters were physical, mental, and emotional.

I had always prayed that others would see Jesus in me. I had prayed that every night before going to sleep for years. Jesus was full of empathy, compassion, and love. He always fought for others. During this struggle,

PAIN WITH POISE

I could no longer pray like I had before the accident. I wondered if it was because trauma was now associated with prayer. I wondered if it was because my body had fought for survival. I wondered if it was because of all the pain and confusion. I just knew I had a different relationship with God.

They say life and skills prepare a leader for a crisis. During my crisis, I, the leader, ended up falling. My communication was suffering. I struggled to function. I succumbed to pain and injuries. My crisis grew into years. As the crisis lengthened, I began falling more and more. While at first, I met each fall with a resolute pick-up, over time, I began running on fumes. I was being emptied by a bad medical team, pain, trauma, endless physical therapy, diminishing hope, opposing legal counsels, trying to maintain jobs, and attempting to function daily. All the while, I could feel the judgmental stares.

In the past, I could work on myself to build myself into a leader using the basic leadership skills. Now, leadership looked different. These days, leadership was about survival. Leadership was about face-contorting pain. Leadership was about being alone. Leadership was about telling the truth while doctors let me suffer.

Leadership became acknowledging that brains were weird, and forgiving myself for each time I failed to live up to my normal living rules and standards. Leadership was cursing. Leadership was trying even if it was a bad idea and failing. Leadership was thinking hell was here to stay. Leadership was suffering in silence, distracting myself, and trying to remain poised until my energy depleted.

PART 1
THE ACCIDENT AND THE AFTERMATH

*The human body is simply
the most beautiful complexity.*

—Daniela Ismerio[1]

1.
PERSPECTIVES

THE CONSCIOUS

CAUTION: The following section may be emotionally distressing.

I had accepted a job to work full-time at a bank. My dad had worked as a bank teller before continuing his successful career. I thought it would be cool to work as a bank teller to explore leadership and obtain my Master's of Business Administration. On May 14, 2018, I drove to my new job's headquarters for training. It was a three-hour drive to an area I had never been. My car was just out of the repair shop due to an issue I had been having with the fuel line. I was thankful to finally have it repaired for the drive and to not have to worry about a car repair with my new job. I finished my first day of training and stayed overnight in the unfamiliar town.

    On my second day of training at the bank's headquarters, I left work chatting with the Human Resources Specialist Sebastian about the day. Sebastian repeatedly asked if I needed to go to the restroom before leaving, but I stated I did not. I was eager to return home and start my new job. Plus, it was drizzling, and I knew the roads would be wet.

    I could feel it, though, and Sebastian stated it later at the hospital. He had felt it, too. There was something in the air, a heavy sense of evil or doom. Something hadn't felt right when I had left Sebastian. Because of this eerie feeling, I sent a text to my mom before I left the bank to let her know I would be returning home soon. Then, I made sure my phone was put away in my driver's side door pocket for a safe, undistracted drive home. While I am always a safe driver, I made a special note to not be "distracted" because of this bad feeling. I decided to play it extremely safe.

• • •

A few minutes passed, and I came to a major intersection. I thought I had just turned out of the driveway of the bank and onto the main road. To my left was a pretty, two-story white house, which was facing acres of farmland. At this intersection, I saw a nicely maintained and very large two-lane road on my right that stretched for miles between the acres of farmland. The farmland had no corn. I had a driveway to my left to enter the farmhouse property, and then immediately after the driveway was another very small road without any painted lines on it, which was my road. My Garmin GPS said to turn left. I turned on my turn signal. I verified my turn on the left and turned. I heard a voice in my car that was not my Garmin say, "Turn right."

Intuition saves your life when you listen to it. Instead, I puzzled at the voice but continued to turn my steering wheel to follow my Garmin.

In that instant, I vividly recall: *I turned my steering wheel to the left.* Then, I heard a sound I later described as a bomb. Then, the left edge of my front windshield filled with gray objects. It was like 9/11. Like a building fell, followed by the silence of people walking away, covered in dust. I saw those gray objects in the corner of my windshield…and then I woke up. I felt nothing. I never knew what was going on, and it was like the time never passed. There was just a bomb. Then nothing.

[Unconscious]

I opened my eyes as I began to regain consciousness. Without moving one muscle, I saw broken glass in the tray under my center console. I was in my driver's seat with my head hanging toward the right. Dazed, I realized I had been in an accident. I attempted to turn my head to the left, but it only would move enough for me to see that my car door was gone. I stared at the metal edge of a white trailer that belonged to a semi-trailer truck.

There was a small space between my car and the trailer. In shock I thought, *I've been hit by a tractor-trailer and I'm still alive!* My next thought was, *Fire!* I was afraid of fire. I was afraid my car would catch on fire and blow up. I was focused on survival.

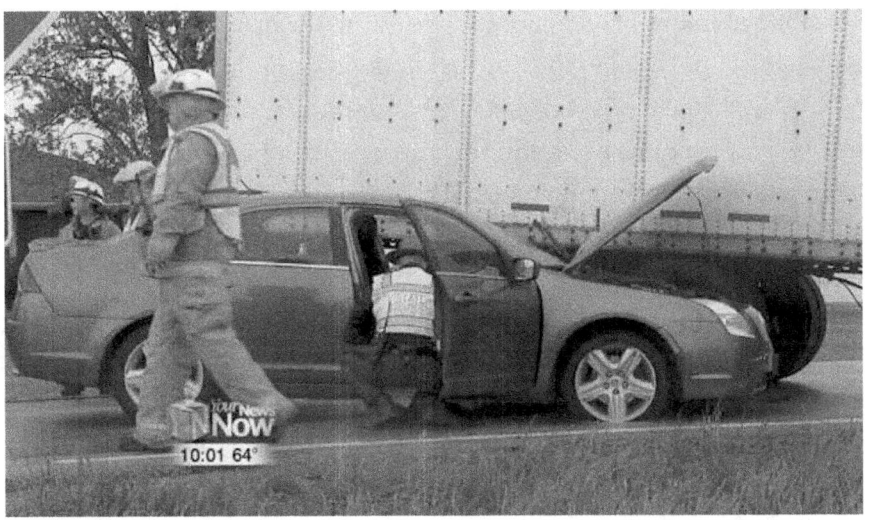

The tractor-trailer accident. Your Hometown Stations. Used by permission.[2]

I assessed the situation. I realized I could not turn my neck left to look at the damage. What I was able to see, though, was enough to realize I could not get out of the car between the car and the trailer. I devised a plan to cross the center console to the passenger seat by staying upright and keeping my spine straight. I prepared to lift a leg.

[Memories Gone]

PAIN WITH POISE

I did make it out of the car through the passenger's side. I don't know how I did it. I have no memory of getting out of the car. I have no memory of anything. I know I had put my seat belt on at the bank. I don't know how I got out of it. I don't remember releasing it.

I somehow found myself outside of the Mercury Milan I'd nicknamed "Cleopatra." I saw a field and a man staring at the right side of the trailer of the 18-wheeler. He seemed so far away from me. Miles and miles away. I wanted to sit on the ground, but I could not get down. I was stumbling blindly. I had no idea where I was. The man saw me and rushed to me to get me back in the car. I sat back down in the passenger seat.

As I sat there, my senses started returning. The silence I was experiencing was the same silence in the movies after a bomb goes off and the person is walking around and can't hear anything, including the ringing. As the silence dissipated, I heard my OnStar® Emergency Services saying I'd been in an accident. I heard my car alarm beeping over and over again. My brain only perceived what was in the car. I don't know anything about my windshield or the view beyond it.

From my right-side view, I saw vehicles pulling up. People were running toward me. A woman arrived and a doctor, dressed in a high white collar like a clergy member, reached my door. Another man arrived and found my cell phone, which was used to call my job. I had the foresight to put the bank's phone number in my cell phone contacts. I was in a very small town, so this bank was also well known by the people arriving. The bank contacted my family.

The shock on everybody's faces terrified me. People stared back at me with looks of sheer horror and panic. I could not imagine what they were seeing. So, I did the scariest thing ever. I pulled my visor mirror down to see what they were seeing. It was not what I was expecting. It was my face with a knot with a slit over my left eye. However, the lack of blood on my face horrified me even more, because I had blood on my hands.

PERSPECTIVES

The blood was not regular blood. It was mixed with shreds of something and was vile. I had never seen anything like it in real life. I knew there was blood somewhere, so I frantically searched for the source of the blood. I checked my mouth for missing and broken teeth. To my shock, they were intact.

My arms were cut and bloodied. My brain was telling me my left ear had been severed from my head. With my left hand, I checked to see if my ear was still attached. It was still attached, to my relief, but I was horrified because I still could not find the source of the blood. I was afraid I had pieces of door impaled in my head. From what had happened, and the looks on everyone's faces, that was the only logical explanation for the blood. I just couldn't find it yet. I had glass in my mouth, and the woman ran back to her car to grab a water bottle. I swished and spit to get the glass and blood out of my mouth.

Then, I looked at the people around me, and I lost it. I was beginning to suffocate. I was trapped. I started screaming and yelling at the people, "Go away!" Reality had hit. The pain was finally hitting. I was in agony. I wanted everything and everyone gone. I wanted to be home in my safe house. I was suffocating and my world was shrinking to being a person in the passenger seat in a car sandwiched between bystanders standing in shock staring at me and a semi-trailer truck.

My body and brain started recognizing the pain. My brain felt indescribable. It felt like it was short-circuiting. I was yelling, "My brain. My brain!" on the inside because it was horrific. It felt like I was going to pass out. I was afraid I would have a seizure. I decided the probability of having a seizure or passing out again was astronomically high from my brain short-circuiting. There was an ill feeling to my brain. It was not the feeling of a migraine or headache or any form of head pain. It didn't feel like brain fog from concussions. It was like I had electricity surging through my brain. I did not know what my brain would do next.

The ambulance arrived. I walked to the stretcher, because I could not sit by that tractor-trailer another second. The paramedics were shoving me back in the car, but I probably would've started attacking people if my arms would've cooperated. A stiff cervical collar was put on me. I will never forget how lifeless my arms were as I laid on that stretcher.

I remember lying on the stretcher as they wheeled me to the ambulance. The paramedics covered my face with a white blanket because it was raining. I wondered if they thought I was dead.

"I'm not dead," I pleaded with them. I was fighting sheer panic and pure terror. The fleeting thought of the horror of being buried alive passed through my mind. As much as I wanted to, I could not move my hands to get the sheet off. Then, my thoughts passed to the bystanders. I was afraid the children would think I was dead. Again, I said, "I'm not dead!" I didn't want one person to think I was dead. I had survived. I was alive. It didn't work. The paramedic was persistent. My face would not get wet under his watch.

In reality, there was a very distinct difference between my memories of the accident and what really happened. I have no memory upon leaving the bank until the time I approached my turn. In the following section, I will describe the multiple perspectives of the accident. These perspectives include the traffic safety report story, pictures, and the discoveries made from the drive in 2020 (see *Stranger in Consciousness Alone* in Chapter 5).

THE TECHNICALITIES OF THE ACCIDENT

I left the bank.

I drove about 15 minutes through a small town which included a stoplight. I have no memory of this town.

A tractor-trailer, also known as a semi-truck or 18-wheeler, was following me too closely. I either never saw or have no memory of this semi. The semi driver swerved left to avoid rear-ending me just when I turned left to access the road to the interstate. The tractor-trailer was hauling 40 tons, or 80,000 pounds, of freight in its trailer. The freight was precisely loaded to full capacity. To save the load, the semi driver then turned right. When he turned right, the front right of the cab truck impacted my driver's side door. My door ripped off while my car went from left to right. As the semi-trailer truck continued moving, the trailer scraped the driver's side of the car for a second impact.

The 18-wheeler ended up in a field with its back wheels at the side of my car, which would have been at least a third impact. The semi-trailer truck did not jackknife because the semi's freight had been precisely loaded to be fully packed. This tight packing actually prevented the load from shifting within the trailer when the truck swerved sharply. From the initial impact, both the front and right front of the cab truck were damaged. The driver of the semi-truck reported injuries but did not need an ambulance. The tractor-trailer driver stated he was not distracted prior to the accident and lost his Class A operating license at the scene.

BY THE PICTURES

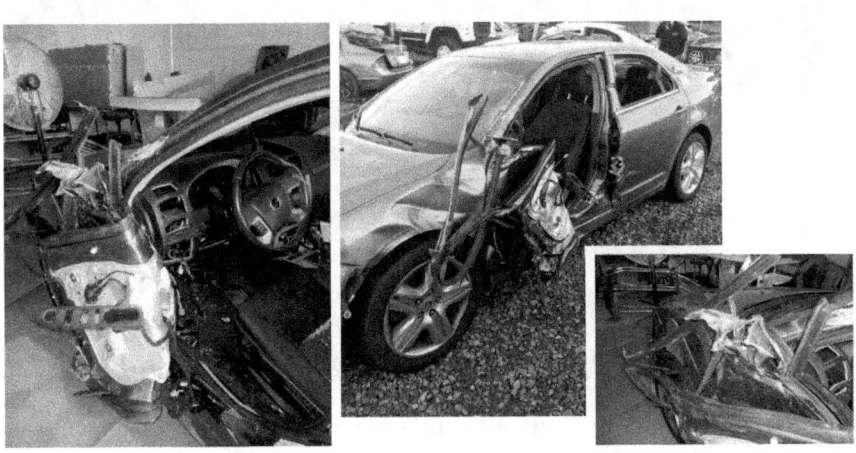

The driver's side door that the tractor-trailer cabin had ripped off upon impact and the twisted, shredded metal that remained of my 2010 Mercury Milan.

PAIN WITH POISE

My driver's side door was ripped off at the lock by the 18-wheeler and peeled forward to the front of the car. The panel of the door was lying on the road. My seat was rotated. The hood was up on my car. The glass was missing from my driver's side rear door. The trailer edge had gouged a line down the side of my car. My front windshield had cracked glass on the left side; it was still intact. The semi-trailer truck had smashed my left front console where my left leg had been. My steering wheel was angled. The steering wheel was also damaged. The worst of the damage was where I had been sitting.

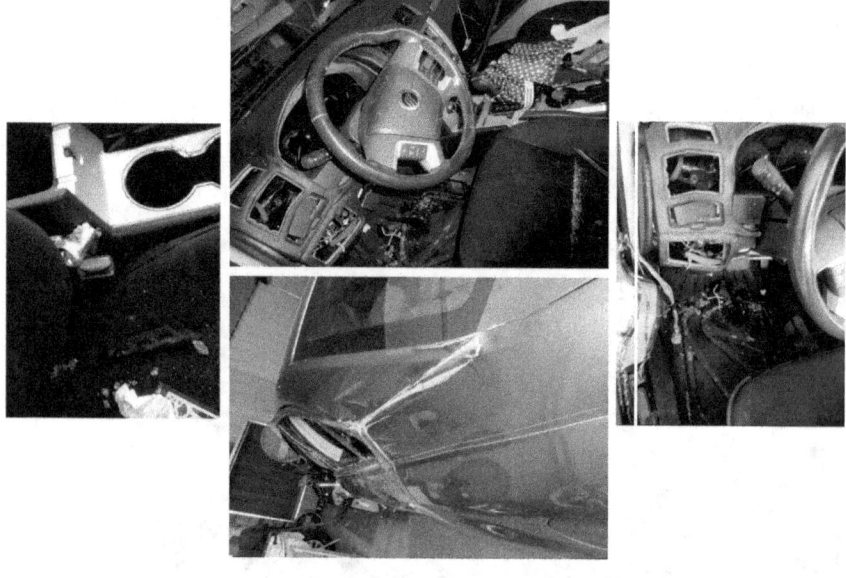

A ripped seltzer can, a bent and twisted steering wheel, a gouged line down the left side of my 2010 Mercury Milan, and a busted driver's side dashboard were all memories from the tractor-trailer's energy on May 15, 2018.

My passenger front axle was broken, and the tire was busted. A seltzer can that had been in my center console was torn in half as if a tornado had ripped through the cabin of my car. Somehow, the glass in my sunroof had remained intact.

PERSPECTIVES

Both vehicles were towed, and the road was closed in both directions for two hours.

POST-ACCIDENT

On the ambulance ride, I had never been in so much pain. Every fiber of my body was screaming. I was shivering and shaking and repeating, "I am so cold." With the IV insertion, I screamed. All my nerves were screaming in my body.

Even with all that nerve pain, the worst pain was in the left side of my jaw. However, it took hours before my body and brain could isolate this body part as pain. I became angry at the doctors because the physician in trauma wanted to show me my ultrasounds while he was doing them. I was not interested, and I was in so much pain. My blood pressure was elevated, and it was elevated for so long, the doctor grew concerned. I learned I had a gash over my left ear that spanned several inches.

I had a chest X-ray, pelvis X-ray, CT scan of my cervical spine and head, and a cervical spine MRI. Before being subjected to X-rays, they ordered a pregnancy test with my bloodwork. If I had been pregnant, they said they would not have been allowed to do one X-ray. I had an excellent trauma nurse. She called me pretty. I felt anything but. I was put on narcotics for my jaw pain as it was the most pronounced pain of every part of my body. That doesn't mean much because I was in a lot of pain everywhere. I was considered for spine surgery as I was told I had a cervical herniation. I was prepared for the surgery and was placed in a room overnight.

One of the weirdest things I remember about my hospital stay was wanting all of my hospital sheets and lots of pillows around my feet and legs in the hospital bed. The nurse at one point tried to remove them and I wouldn't let her. The blankets and pillows had to stay there until I left. I think it was a safety cocoon that mimicked how my legs were kept safe by my car cabin from the semi-truck. In addition, my room had to stay

PAIN WITH POISE

cold. I woke up at one point during the night stuck in a hard neck brace in a warm room, feeling like I was suffocating. Once I got the room cold again, I was fine.

This hospital wouldn't give me my anti-epileptics, so I had to take them from my overnight bag. Thankfully, the state trooper had brought some of my stuff, and the bank employee salvaged the rest of my personal belongings from my car. I wasn't going to have a seizure, so since the hospital kept forgetting and the hospital medications are really expensive, I took my own medications.

It was determined surgery could wait, and I was released on orders to see my family physician and a spine surgeon. At discharge, my mom asked the nurse what to expect. The nurse replied, "Post-traumatic stress disorder," and left. Upon being released from the hospital, I began to learn the extent of my injuries. I had been on bed rest during my hospital stay. At the time, I was extremely disconnected from reality. I thought my car was fine. I had seen some pictures, and I thought my car just needed a new door.

Stoically, I thought I could walk out of the hospital. I wasn't paralyzed and I wanted to use my legs. However, the nurses refused to let me. They said I would never make it down. I thought this was weird. I was in shape! I obliged them. I went down in a wheelchair. When I got into my parents' car, the man who took me down realized I was the person on the news the night before. The tractor-trailer motor vehicle accident that involved my car was on the news and in the newspaper. It had shut the road down for 4 hours during rush hour. The 18-wheeler had to be towed. When the man discovered who I was, he reached his hand out to shake my hand. I'll never forget it. I'd survived and he got to meet me and I got to meet him. I was alive. My parents took me to Bob Evans to eat.

Then we had a two-hour drive. I yelled at my dad the whole ride home over his driving. I had emotional trauma already. I had so much anxiety I could've puked. I wanted to drive. Nobody was able to drive as cautiously or as safe as me anymore. If we were in a wreck, it could only be my fault.

2.
THE FIRST YEAR OF PHYSICAL SUFFERING

Immediately after the accident, I began the process of reflecting upon what happened and trying to accept it. I began the process of cleanup, trying to heal, and evolving into a new person. I had a mental picture and plan to prepare for the therapies and the challenges. As a marathon runner, I had taken pride in running through pain. I smiled and cheered, and all my pictures showed exactly what I was: a poised woman. All my life I had been genuinely poised. Even when I failed my first-year oral exam and dropped my head in defeat, I had remained poised.

I realized my sunglasses were missing. They had been ripped off my head during the accident. I surmised they were still at the accident scene. I asked the bank's corporate HR if they could look for my sunglasses. They were only 10 minutes away from the accident scene. I was 1.5 hours away. The HR manager gave an adamant no. That irrationally angered me.

On the way home from the hospital, I had my parents drop me off at the grocery store. I needed to pick up three things. I had been placed on a 10-pound weight restriction. My three items were supposed to be easy to carry, yet I found myself huffing and puffing to the sidewalk to meet my parents. My heart was racing from the exertion. That was the first time I went, "Whoa." I started wondering what really did happen to me. What was really wrong with me? I started to get more concerned that this was more than a simple injury. It was like the tractor-trailer had sucked the life out of me. For perspective, the day before the accident, I could have worked over 9 hours at Kohl's, another one of my employers, squatting, lifting, hauling, and pushing carts loaded down with merchandise without huffing. I could no longer walk without huffing because of a semi-trailer truck.

Because I wanted to process the accident alone, I sent my parents home. I was used to living by myself. I was not in the mood to have people around. I could drive. I could buy food. I could sleep. We quickly learned I could not be hugged. I could have no squeezing of the upper body. Instead, my parents just lightly acted like they were hugging me. I was aware of trauma and injuries and pain. I was mentally prepared to beat it. However, I could not have been more unprepared.

The first week, I was alive, and I could walk. That's all that mattered. I was still me. I was not paralyzed. I sat there on my couch, sorting through things. I still followed the old rules: no narcotics. I refused to take any narcotics that first week.

The second week, I visited my family physician. She allowed me to start doing some more of my normal routine with some mild stretches. I went home. With two hands planted on the floor, I pushed up from my stomach. To my horror, it felt like my shoulder blades had crossed over my spine. I felt the contortion like a horror show. When I sat up, it was like all my parts slid back into position.

I sobbed in terror. This feeling happened only once, however, it signaled that I had a lot of physical damage in my back.

This time I finally lost it. I began to lose my poise. The idea of going to the emergency room or urgent care never registered. In fact, I went almost 24 hours before something inside of me finally said I needed to call my doctor. There was something about the shock of my back humping that made my brain begin to wake up to the reality of my semi-truck injuries.

I called my family physician and talked to the nurse the next day. I still had my narcotic prescription from the hospital because I had refused to fill it. I didn't want to take narcotics! But now, my back had deformed and hunched and crisscrossed. I needed narcotics.

I went to the pharmacy to see if they would fill my prescription from

THE FIRST YEAR OF PHYSICAL SUFFERING

the hospital. Everybody at my regular pharmacy felt bad for me, because I had never filled narcotics my whole life. However, they could not because it was an expired prescription note. I was delirious. I called the hospital where I had the accident to see if I could get a new prescription written. I called my family physician and talked to the nurse. I don't even remember what she said, but I said I wanted narcotics. She knew my complaint was legit as she didn't hang up on me when I asked for narcotics. Yet, she was not cooperating, so I finally said, "*You* get hit by a tractor-trailer." I blocked the physician's number on my phone. However, before I could block her, the nurse had left a voicemail to go to urgent care. I was livid. They were my family physician for 14 years. They knew me. They were supposed to see me.

I was in week two of my recovery. The horrors were just starting. I thought I was lucky when I left the hospital.

As the weeks went by, I learned I was unable to clean. My upright vacuum was lightweight and easy to use. However, I couldn't get it up the stairs. I couldn't even vacuum downstairs. Quite frankly, I couldn't vacuum. Vacuuming requires twisting. I considered buying a robot vacuum cleaner, but finances were really tight, so I bought a handheld vacuum. I decided it was lightweight enough and small enough that I could actually use it to vacuum dirt off the floor.

I quickly realized I also couldn't lift my Crock-Pot to cook food. I was forced to switch to freezer meals and other pre-packaged foods. After the accident, I couldn't wash dishes well because my sink was too deep. I wasn't allowed to lean over since that meant I would bend my spine. Extending my arms to clean also involved pain. I also had issues loading and unloading my dishwasher. The list of basic tasks I couldn't complete was getting longer by the day—and my living conditions reflected this.

Every great once in a while, my mom was able to help. Yet, I was starting to live in filth. I didn't have the finances for a housekeeper during my recovery. I was starting to get frustrated by the degree of uncleanliness. In comparison, I used to scrub weekly. The rest of my family lived hours away as well. I was forced to adapt to living conditions that were less clean than I wanted and less clean than I thought was healthy for any human.

My bed became an excruciating place to lay my body down. Before the accident, my bed felt like a cloud, and I never had an ache getting out of bed. After the accident, I felt like I was being poked by nails all over. There was no comfortable position, and the lower thoracic region on my left side hurt so bad I could not sleep on my left side. For weeks, I endured night after night of deep, guttural, involuntary moans when I crawled into bed. The thoracic cramps were pure agony, and I couldn't move to alleviate the pain. I lay there like a dead person until it passed. Thankfully, the cramps went away after a few weeks.

Every morning and every night I had to brace myself for getting into and out of bed. I would brace and roll and let everything settle before attempting the next body roll. When I rolled, it was like I could feel my spine waving, and I was a noodle. My whole body was completely unstable, with needle-like pain being seared into my body. This continued for several minutes of pure agony until I finally was able to somehow get my feet on the floor to get out of bed.

In addition, I realized what it required to change bedding on a bed. Those sheets got changed, but I judged my healing by sheet-changing over the next few years. I went weeks without changing sheets. With the body I had post-tractor trailer, changing sheets became an agonizing workout. Plus, I was not supposed to bend my spine. Sometimes, my sheets just didn't get changed.

I struggled pushing grocery carts at the store, and learned I could barely load them. The worst was turning the grocery cart; it required abdominal strength, and I no longer had any, so I felt pain in my back. I was forced to stop using a grocery cart, and I shopped for only what I could carry. I huffed and puffed. It was awkward and painful.

THE FIRST YEAR OF PHYSICAL SUFFERING

I couldn't put my shoes on without horrendous pain. I had to sit on the bed to put on both pants and shoes. Getting dressed for work required bracing my whole body and brain for the onslaught of pain that would ensue. I could no longer wear heels. Fixing my hair was awful, because I had to raise my arms.

I also couldn't carry my purse, because it was too heavy. I just carried my wallet. Three years after the accident, I still couldn't carry my purse or wear a crossbody purse. By year four, I was able to carry a purse again as I had successfully started rebuilding my core. I had to give up my new favorite chunky black necklace. It was very heavy and was too much weight for my injured and weak neck muscles. I was finally able to wear it five years later.

Taking the stairs was horrible. Both directions were awful, and I would have to take the stairs one at a time. One foot up, then the other. Two feet on the same step. Then, I would attempt the next step. This continued for quite a while.

Getting into a car was horrifically painful, and shutting the door required bracing myself for the waves of pain. The pain wasn't just in my back. It was in my abdomen and legs. Then, of course, getting out was just as bad. I would twist in the seat to face outward prior to standing up. It was exasperating.

Sitting on the couch to watch TV was painful. Sitting on a chair hurt. Existing hurt. Existing felt like needles were being shoved in me or maybe worse, nails. I felt like a thick rubber band that had lost all its elasticity. I couldn't bend, twist, or rotate. I hurt reclining. I hurt sitting up. It hurt if my mom rubbed my feet. It hurt if my mom rubbed my back. Strangely, it didn't hurt where she touched them. It hurt in my head. The pain was like a searing white numbness in my head.

My blood pressure would soar from pain the first couple of years. At doctor appointments, my blood pressure was consistently elevated for me even though it was still within an acceptable level to not need blood pressure medications. Thankfully, my Ohio Bureau of Workers' Compensation (BWC) nurse would comment on it, and did consider it related to pain. Some doctors ignore little things like this, but they are vital to my personal health. After a couple of years, my blood pressure returned to normal. However, this discrepancy meant something was wrong. To me, it meant I was in too much pain. I even gave up coffee due to the tingling pain I'd feel from the caffeine.

If a person lightly tapped me, it would cause pain in my back and up my neck and down my legs because I could not adjust. I had no core stability. Also, I could not tap anything without enduring pain in my back and neck.

3.
ENERGY, FORCE, AND INTERCONNECTEDNESS

Injuries sustained in an accident are directly correlated to the energy involved in the accident, and there was a lot of energy involved in my accident. Even though there were other things involved like brakes, seat belts, and air bags to save my life, energy goes through them all. Those things can only do so much and can still cause damage. This is a simple physics and accident breakdown of why high-impact injuries may be so unusual and so unexpectedly severe.

Air bags reduce the movement of the body and organs. My car had front and side air bags for the driver, front and side air bags for the passenger, and side air bags for the backseat passengers. These air bags are designed to only deploy at certain angles. According to the state trooper, my accident did not happen at one of those angles. Therefore, my air bags did not deploy. Since mine did not deploy, my body endured the maximum force to which it was subjected.

I was wearing my seat belt at the time of the accident, even though I had no bruising from a seat belt. I had a few hypotheses about the lack of bruising. My driver's seat in my car was reclined slightly back for ergonomic driving. This was a recommendation from a chiropractor. Because I am petite and short waisted, I sit upright when I am making turns so I am able to see clearly. This means the shoulder belt at impact would have been loose instead of tightly binding me against the car seat. My first hypothesis was the loose shoulder belt did not impact my torso to cause bruising or injury. My second hypothesis was the impact was from the side causing

PAIN WITH POISE

my body to shift sideways with the loose shoulder belt. Another hypothesis was that I fought briefly before losing consciousness, so my arms were braced against the steering wheel. The combined loose shoulder belt and my arms braced against the steering wheel prevented belt injury. A fourth hypothesis was that I don't bruise easily. My final hypothesis was I saw the 18-wheeler and in my last attempt to save my life, I unbuckled my seat belt to dive for safety but never left my seat.

In the resource section at the end of this book, I discuss the physics and details of the accident in detail.

The energy from the tractor-trailer soaked into my body. The bad energy soaks into a driver's energy and disrupts it at impact—the tiny little ruptures, the little wrinkles, the broken fibers, the malfunctioning neuron pathways, and the nerves and cells absorbing the kinetic energy from the impact. I became a disrupted energy field in need of repair.

Immediately after my accident, I learned there was a lot wrong with my body. As time passed and I began to increase activity, I really learned the true extent of the destruction. The longer rehabilitation progressed, the more I realized it wasn't working. This suggested to me that my injuries were worse than initially believed. When I thought back to that fateful day in 2018, I began hypothesizing what may have happened to my body. I had absorbed a lot of energy in that 18-wheeler accident that a human was not designed to absorb. As I had absorbed the energy of the semi-trailer truck it had become a part of me. The bad energy that my body was not designed to handle resulted in shredded and damaged cells. I had to heal my body and I had to do so by thinking about the energy that had caused it injury and by envisioning all my body parts.

The human body consists of muscles, joints, and the fascial system—about 650 muscles and 360 joints, to be exact. The brain, nerves, and skeletal muscles comprise the neuromuscular system.[1] A band of connective tissue, called fascia, holds the body together. These bands of tissue wrap around every organ, blood vessel, bone, nerve fiber, and muscle to

ENERGY, FORCE, AND INTERCONNECTEDNESS

hold them in position.[2] In one instant, all of these parts of my body were impacted by a peak impact force equivalent to 18.129 MN[3] when my car and I were hit by a fully loaded tractor-trailer. Sadly, I wasn't hit just once. While I don't know how many times my car was impacted by the semi-trailer truck, I knew each additional hit further damaged already damaged muscle and nerves.

It would be years before I would learn the true extent of my injuries and how seriously I was hurt. However, I began applying my knowledge of science at my first doctor's appointment when I decided I was given bad advice. When I chose to not follow a doctor's advice, I did so because I knew what had hit me. My common sense and education told my brain to prepare. I felt the way I did for a reason. Something was very wrong.

I had not been hit by a football, or a car. I had been hit *by a tractor-trailer*. The numbers told me the different stories. This was an extreme impact force injury. To heal, I began a journey following my own intuition, education, and knowledge.

THE NEW CONSCIOUSNESS OF THE INTERNAL BODY

The Spine

My spine surgeon wanted me to immobilize my spine in case it contained a fracture that had been missed. This was important because he stated I had been hit by a semi-truck, and there could be a hairline fracture in the cervical spine or other parts of the spine. I needed additional imaging. I was given specific neck stretches to perform. My spine surgeon said there was to be no movement of my neck from a forward to backward position, but instead I should use an ear-to-shoulder stretch with no twisting motion. This contradicted my family physician's suggestion of stretching my neck with a forward and backward motion.

Some things I reported to my physicians were that my spine felt like it was a metal rod from neck to lumbar. It also felt like my spine was a stack of bricks at times. It would feel like this for months. During this time, I still didn't believe my doctors when they said that my spinal cord was okay. I had so many things wrong with me that I was sure my spinal cord was irritated or something. The problem was, we had to wait on a full body scan, and most facilities do not have these. In fact, the hospital I had been in didn't have one.

Therefore, I lived, waiting in terror, thinking I had a spine fracture. Thankfully, I did not have a fractured spine and my spine surgeon wanted to wait to see if my acute cervical herniation would heal with rehabilitation. I was then transferred for physical therapy.

The Neurological System

Everyday responsibilities of nerves include making us aware of sensations such as pain, and engaging muscles so we can move, like when a doctor hits a knee with a doctor's plexor. Nerves carry electrical impulses between the brain and body via neurons. These neurons send signals along a pathway or a network of neurons so the brain can communicate with other parts of the body.[4] After the semi-trailer truck accident, I learned what nerves could do. In short, my neuron pathways were wonky. They were doing crazy things.

Within a few weeks of the accident, I was in the shower before work one morning, when I closed my eyes and I could not get them to reopen. I was frozen in place, paralyzed by horror. I had to pry my eyelids open. That event happened only once.

I had two episodes where I was standing and had a violent upper body whip. I was walking through the kitchen one night and my spine curled violently, and I whipped forward from the waist. My spine curled on me like I was wrapped around an exercise ball. My arms went forward

ENERGY, FORCE, AND INTERCONNECTEDNESS

and my hands rotated at the wrists. The scariest part was that my arms didn't twitch. My arms were not involved in the movement. My legs were not involved. It was not like I jumped. I stayed planted. My wrists and hands moved without moving my arms. It was a terrifying, abnormal movement.

I now believe my body was reliving the violent impact of the 18-wheeler. Perhaps upon impact, my hands shook against the steering wheel and my arms were locked stiff. When my upper body whipped weeks after the accident, it was so violent that I was afraid I would throw myself across the room.

My physical medicine and rehabilitation (PM&R) doctor suggested it was nerve-related. I had no idea what he was talking about. He then just sat there and stared at me. He told me nothing about what to do or how to stop it. He told me nothing about how to prevent my fear that it would happen again. He didn't prescribe medications. He did nothing. When I started thinking about it over the years, I realized nerves could take a person over like an epileptic seizure. In that second, a person had no control.

Most people have had random toe twitches, finger twitches, or annoying eye twitches. I had never experienced anything of this magnitude, though. That moment was when I realized the power of the neuron pathway.

I suffered from a pinched nerve that made it hard to move or bend. While it was a low-grade pain compared to the other searing pain, I was still in agony from it. This pain was not from sciatica, and I wasn't diagnosed with the appropriate nerve pain until months later. Josh Murphy, D.C., at Murphy Chiropractic & Performance Center (MCPC), diagnosed me with a pinched femoral nerve in 2019. The pain in my buttocks was from the femoral nerve, and it went all the way down the inside of my leg from the back of my buttocks.

I also had really bad numbness and tingling in my right hand. While I had some really minor issues of tingling in my right hand prior to the accident, it was magnitudes different after the accident. It was almost my whole hand that was numb. This experience taught me that when you have preexisting symptoms, doctors can miss new issues.

My eyes would even rotate in place. These eye rotations were not eye rolls. I could only surmise they were neurological. They were not like eye rolls from seizures. It was usually the moment when superhuman strength or power overcame me. It could have even been related to my concussion. It could have been from nerve irritability from whiplash or even my cranial nerves. Thankfully, these episodes decreased over time.

Part of my left arm gave me some issues—I figured it was nerve pain. The pain was in the center of my tricep. I had nerve issues in my jaw and teeth. At the time, I swore the nerve was connected and traveled up to my arm to my teeth. My local neurologist assured me nerve pain only traveled down. I wasn't so sure. If I pressed my arm, I could feel the nerves in my teeth. I swore tractor-trailers created a new pattern within the body. An electromyography also showed some nerve irritability in my left elbow. In 2024, Active Edge Chiropractic & Functional Medicine (Active Edge) shifted focus to look at this spot. The fascia was riddled with scar tissue and made snap and crackle sounds while the chiropractic assistant worked it out.

One day I reported to my first physical therapists that my legs felt like tree trunks. They felt fat and stubby. They didn't feel like legs. I was informed it was due to nerve irritability. So was the sensation of water (or blood, as I'd also feared) running down my upper back.

I screamed a lot during the early phase of my recovery. A lot of that was due to nerve pain. While we all have nerves that tell us when things hurt, nerve pain is particularly brutal.

I endured stabbing pain. I endured searing pain. I endured raw pain. I also learned about gravel-like pain, which was nauseating, laced with spasms and muscle cramps. I also experienced the equivalent of a sunburn all over my body. This pain went straight to the brain.

ENERGY, FORCE, AND INTERCONNECTEDNESS

Early on, the pain would take me over and I would start screaming or being brash and loud or yell. It was for this reason I was thankful I did not live in an apartment. I was unable to hide the truth of the hell I was enduring from people. The worst part was that I was not able to recognize this nerve pain as nerve pain. This is why I call it a quiet, silent pain—and sensory overload pain. It was both a covert and overt pain. It was not just a burning or tingling or sharp pain.

Nerve pain is something that my brain recognized but my consciousness and knowledge could not.

For example, I was not consciously aware I was in pain, because it wasn't like a pinched nerve. However, if I stubbed my toe or hit my shin, I was in agony that was much greater than a stubbed toe should produce. It went straight to my brain, and I would see flashing lights. I began explaining it to doctors as feeling like I had been set on fire.

I also could feel my teeth in a way that I never had before. I didn't have a cavity. I had a full dental exam and my mouth was still perfectly healthy, with no need for dental work. It was a miracle that I had no fractured jaw. This was a separate issue from the nerve issues in the left side of my torso connected to my left arm. The nerves in my teeth hurt, and I complained I could feel my skeletal structure. Since nerves are in bone, I believed the nerves in my bone were also irritated by the tractor-trailer impact.

After the accident, I was horrified to periodically see all my fingers and half my palm go white and numb on my right hand. While I have Raynaud's phenomenon,[5] it's always been very mild. This was the worst episode of Raynaud's phenomena triggered yet. The semi-truck had really upset my body, and my neurological system was greatly overreacting to all kinds of stimuli.

I was constantly nauseated from the pain. My brain was in zombie land, and it felt as if my nerves had been stretched and shredded. I was not able to focus or have clear vision. I was unable to handle any additional stress. This continued for years.

PAIN WITH POISE

The Rest of the Human Body

My injuries weren't limited to the spine and brain. I also had pain in my right groin that extended all the way along my lower pelvis to my anus. There was something along my right buttocks that felt wrong. My right leg was rotated severely outward, and any attempt to rotate it forward failed. When I say severe, my leg appeared to be rotated outward 45 degrees. However, nobody measured the angle. I could only imagine my right leg had almost been severed in the accident.

In one of the stranger sensations after the accident, I felt like my butt was way out in front of the rest of my body. Anatomically, I knew where it actually was. It was like a form of dissociation. I had no connection to this part of my body from a brain standpoint. It felt how I imagine it would feel to be an amputee having phantom sensations. This part of my body—pivotal for moving around the world—felt as though it was positioned well out in front of me. It was totally disorienting.

My major complaint in trauma was my left jaw. It hurt in a way I could not describe. For weeks and months after the wreck, I swore my face looked different on that side every time I saw myself. I would stand there and stare and stare and stare trying to decide if the reflection was my real face or my mind playing tricks on me. I couldn't look at myself in the mirror anymore, because it bothered me so much.

I suffered from muscle spasms in the face, neck, and back. The underlying pain was a searing white pain or a gravel-inducing pain with nausea. At other times, I endured chest pain that made it hard to breathe, along with arm twitches and extreme face pain. My face would contort, and my tongue behaved as a possessed muscle moving inside my mouth. I was informed by my neurologist that this was due to my weak neck muscles. However, I literally had sensations of wanting to spit it out of my mouth.

I had a gash over my left ear, which was the side the tractor-trailer impacted. I was stunned and thankful at the lack of scarring—I ended up with just a single scar underneath my hair and one on my lip. During recovery, I had a bump with a slit over my left eye, and a soccer ball-sized bruise on the outside of my left knee. Since the windows on the left side exploded into tiny pieces, I had tiny glass cuts all over my arms and lips. One cut left a scar on my lip. However, it was nothing that stuck out. I was really lucky. I don't know why my face was spared, but it was.

Over the next couple of months, my menstrual cycle slowly vanished. About 5 to 6 months after the accident, I visited my gynecologist. She told me she believed it was due to trauma from the accident. Quite simply, the 18-wheeler had tried to split me in half at the groin, like a wishbone at Thanksgiving. My other doctors didn't understand this. My doctors sent me to work like this. I'm thankful for my amazing gynecologist.

Sadly, my injuries and chronic pain have made it unlikely that I will ever be pregnant. My chiropractor discussed how the body pulls nutrients and energy from organs not considered vital to heal other body parts. This was a topic even in 2020 as my body was still under so much stress from trying to rehab.

I woke up with red eyes one day soon after the accident. It was really concerning. I had never had this issue before, even when I was tired or had allergies. I mentioned this when I saw my physical therapist. I still don't know what caused the redness. It was as if the tractor-trailer had given me a new body.

The Concussion

I thought about all the money that had been used to educate and train my brain since I was born, maybe even before I was born. I decided it was a million-dollar brain if I could calculate all the money the government, my parents, and companies had invested in it. For example, my brain developed from books, music, and public school teachers. It developed from Sunday school teachers, the Bible, and my family. My brain absorbed information from the television, movies, and the radio. It digested the basics of running a farm, such as planting seeds and canning, from my family who had acres of farmland. One day, my brain even figured out how to prove a trigonometric identity that stumped my own professor.

Then, I went to graduate school. My brain learned even more. In my professional career, my brain gained knowledge in chemistry, physics, biochemistry, and engineering. My brain developed its emotional and cultural intelligence using relationship building in several ways—online, professionally, and in my marriage. I invested in my million-dollar brain with healthy foods and exercise. I chose a lower stress life. I chose to avoid situations where I would be emotionally abused. I definitely avoided situations where I would be physically abused. When something is worth a million dollars, it is precious. I had to take care of it.

But let's take a step back for a moment. The brain regulates the body so a person can live. If a person didn't have a brain, that person would die. If a person had a brain transplant, they would lose their memories. The brain regulates a person's breathing, blood pressure, heart rate, and swallowing. It controls how a person responds during a stressful situation. It coordinates movements of the eyes and face, balance, hearing, as well as sensations of the face. It controls eyelid opening and closing, neck and shoulder muscles, and even the tongue. It controls eating, sexual behavior, and sleeping. Body temperature, emotions, hormone secretion and movement are all regulated by the brain as well. Remembering new information, recalling information, recognizing human faces or objects, and speech function and spatial processing are all responsibilities of the brain.[6]

Without the brain fully functioning, we have the potential to suffer greatly. For all of these reasons, a person needs his brain to be healthy. Plus, it needs to be injury-free for a person's future to be their best future. I loved myself and who I had become. I greatly valued my brain, because it was the only reason I was who I had become.

ENERGY, FORCE, AND INTERCONNECTEDNESS

And then, when that million-dollar brain was knocked unconscious by a tractor-trailer, confusion immediately started. When I arrived at the hospital, I remembered one pivotal question asked by the doctor. "Did you lose consciousness?" I stated the only thing I knew. "I don't remember the accident." I thought that meant I had lost consciousness. Sebastian, the HR specialist from the bank, had even overheard my answer. They never asked any clarifying questions. For whatever reason, they put down "no loss of consciousness," which was the exact opposite of what I meant. In fact, when I stated the very same thing to my family doctor for my follow-up visit, she stated that I had lost consciousness. I chose to use her advice. She advised two hours of daily rest to "watch the birds" for brain healing.

Through the years after the accident, I started to notice additional brain deficits. In high school, I had to memorize the Gettysburg Address. For decades, I would just spontaneously recite, "four score and seven years ago,"[7] for no reason. While I still knew a score was 20 years, after I was hit by a semi-trailer truck, I forgot this statement. I also forgot the Pledge of Allegiance. I knew certain parts of it. However, I couldn't make it all the way through without help. In 2021, I finally made myself re-memorize it.

The same thing happened with Bible verses I had memorized, including my favorite Bible verse. I had memory blocks even to my favorite Bible verse, Proverbs 3:5-6. I stumbled over words or was uncertain of the next word. In addition, I learned something else. If I tried to do an internal monologue, the wrong words would jumble up the sentence I was thinking. However, saying the sentence out loud usually helped.

I had a strange issue. My brain was not fully functioning, and I was walking around like a zombie. I looked normal and acted basically normal, but I was far from it. I could name the current president, but I had a lot of deficits. An estimated 5.3 million people in the United States and 500,000 people in Canada suffer from long-term effects from traumatic brain injuries.[8] I was wondered if I was done forever.

PAIN WITH POISE

As the doctor in trauma misunderstood me and wrote that I did not lose consciousness, this gave BWC a lot of power. While my family physician had diagnosed me with a concussion with loss of consciousness at my first follow-up, it didn't matter. Even if I had not lost consciousness, I still had a knot over my left eye and a gash over my left ear. I was shocked I was not given a diagnosis of a concussion in the trauma unit.

According to the Glasgow Coma Scale (GCS), I had a traumatic brain injury (TBI). The GCS is best for diagnosing a TBI, but not determining the recovery outcome, as it fails to accurately access the outcome of a mild traumatic brain injury. I had also lost consciousness. Loss of consciousness is also associated with a small percentage of concussions.[9] I also had memory loss, even if I did not know this until years later. That period of memory has never returned.

While my family physician immediately diagnosed me with a concussion, she no longer wanted to handle my appointments related to the accident, because she said it was supposed to be billed under BWC. I suffered greatly at her neglect, because she was wrong. I had no other doctor yet.

Getting a BWC doctor required a lot of steps. Let's pause and consider the insurance process I was navigating in Ohio. I was uninsured when the semi-trailer hit me. My insurance at the bank was still in its probationary period. I was being paid by the bank for the commute when the accident happened, so the bank's HR informed me I would be using BWC for insurance. I was skeptical. They seemed positive.

I immediately found a personal injury attorney to handle my personal injury case, and the firm recommended their BWC attorney to represent me in the BWC case. My personal injury attorney was not very pleased about the idea of opening a BWC claim. However, the partner of the firm thought this was the best arrangement for me since I was uninsured. Therefore, I obliged, and we began the process of opening a BWC claim.

My employer initially stated they would cover everything with "no fight." I received the first managed care organization's (MCO) initial claim

ENERGY, FORCE, AND INTERCONNECTEDNESS

letter in the mail. The MCO was opened under three separate body parts: my neck, my chest, and my pelvis. I even talked to an MCO representative on the phone. Then, the bank switched MCOs. The second MCO required an Ohio Industrial Commission (IC) hearing to open a claim.

To open a BWC claim, my BWC attorney and I had to go to the IC for a hearing. The bank had a MCO representative attend the hearing. The bank's Human Resources department had the authority to tell the MCO to fight or not fight a claim. A hearing officer at the IC heard all claims to determine if they were approved or denied.

My BWC attorney's main goal was to open a claim for a body part. He started with the neck, because we had imaging. He said we could later add more claims. The MCO representative, who was female, said the employer was not fighting the claim. The IC hearing officer, who was female, approved the claim for my neck only. I was finally able to get a primary care doctor within the BWC network.

This was the only time they did not fight. Later, the BWC family doctor referred me to a BWC neurologist for a non-concussion diagnosis. When I saw him, he diagnosed me with a concussion from the accident just like my family doctor. This BWC neurologist wanted me to have additional treatments for the concussion. However, my BWC family doctor was not interested in filling out the paperwork.

When I began seeing a new BWC family doctor, he filled out the paperwork for a new claim for a concussion. The MCO representative continued to fight brutally. The MCO found out about an old concussion and made up that I was still suffering from my old concussion. I'm not really sure how this happened. I was really angry, because I needed care for my head. Concussions are very dangerous. If I had a broken finger that had healed and had broken it again in the accident, I believe the MCO would have called it a pre-existing condition. The MCO representative was that evil. It was for this reason I could no longer speak to the bank. The IC refused to rule that I had a concussion, which meant I would have had no medical coverage for my concussion if I had still been uninsured.

As I now had medical insurance through Kohl's, I began seeing doctors and physical therapists using my own insurance. However, copays and deductibles were things that were not supposed to be my responsibility from a concussion sustained in an accident when on work time. I wanted my concussion covered by BWC.

After this hearing, I reported the MCO representative. His manager was really nice and asked if I wanted him removed from my case. I also side-eyed those who worked for the bank's Human Resources department and wondered what was wrong with them. That was as cruel and heartless as a person could get. I do wonder if they hated me. If in reading, one finds this emotional, it's because it is. Even after decades of research, a concussion is still an invisible illness, which can cause extreme disruption in a person's social and professional life. It affects one's cognitive, emotional, sensory, and motor functions.[10] A person can greatly suffer for life due to a concussion. Getting adequate diagnosis, treatment, and compensation for a concussion matters.

I still don't know how the MCO got access to previous medical records that said I had a previous concussion in my lifetime. I'm really sort of weirded out by how they were able to access my medical records in the first place. I was aghast at what happened. The MCO representative not only convinced the hearing officer a concussion was a pre-existing condition, but succeeded at convincing the hearing officer my previous concussion meant it was impossible to ever sustain a second concussion. This flawed logic meant any new concussion I sustained, including the head injury from the tractor-trailer accident, could only occur in the same area of the brain as my prior concussion. This was preposterous logic. A concussion can occur in any region of the brain, which is why each concussion is unique. It seemed to me the MCO representative was hoping to convince the hearing officer a concussion caused permanent brain damage or it was a whole brain injury—but that is a diffuse axonal brain injury which results in coma.[11]

ENERGY, FORCE, AND INTERCONNECTEDNESS

READING AND WRITING

To show the difference in the functioning of my brain, I selected a couple of resumes. My resumes in 2017 were written without needing any professional advice. In fact, my first resume written post- Chemical Abstracts Service got me a second round interview into the Washington, D.C., region within days of writing it. It was in my specialty. I just chose a different journey. In the meantime, I discovered I could write an outstanding curriculum vitae, which was several pages long. This curriculum vitae got me two adjunct professor positions.

After the accident, I struggled to write a resume. I was sending out resumes with grammatically incorrect sentences and structuring. I would consistently cut sentences so my sentences ended early. Other times, I would write a sentence with no subject or with no verb, for example. To make matters worse, I didn't even realize this error until years later when my brain was finally able to register the error.

I was horrified, because it was not acceptable. I had been writing since I was young and had even won several awards. Before the accident, I had been coached to perfection, or close to it, for one reason—perfection led to success. While I didn't consider myself a perfectionist—my house had items out of position and my clothes were never folded—perfection had been necessary in my collegiate and professional world. Plus, my professional world was still raising the bar higher.

When it came to writing, it was a task that required little effort to yield perfect and pleasing results. This was why I enjoyed writing before the accident. I was used to being able to quickly scan something and catch errors and quickly resolve them. I was used to working for a publisher. Now, I just saw garble. I was practically dyslexic. In addition, I was suffering from pain and migraines. This compounded the issue. I could no longer quickly write a resume. I could no longer appropriately write using the correct verb tense. In fact, I could not proofread. I could no longer see

PAIN WITH POISE

errors. I did not see missing periods. I did not see incomplete sentences. It took a few years before I realized I was writing in a weird way.

While healing from my concussion, there were good days and bad days. Even after a lot of things began to heal, I still had bad days when I would write horrific resumes and think they read okay. On bad days, I couldn't function. It was like day one all over again. I would write like a robot first learning how to speak and write. It was almost stunted. Incorrect words were inserted. Even now, I have to double- and triple-check my work for the most simplistic of sentences.

I wrote to a company one day advocating for a cause. I received an email back from one of the executive customer service representatives. There were a few errors in his email. I paused. It was imperfect. An executive had an imperfect email—it gave me hope. Perhaps he was a former football player who had sustained a concussion. I was pleased his company didn't judge his imperfections. He inspired me. I still think of him and his email. It's him and companies like his who hire imperfect humans and let them work that inspire this new imperfect me to continue with my dreams. They let them achieve dreams.

It was difficult to visualize a paragraph and remember thoughts or ideas to apply those in a structured essay. I also had difficulty determining how I wanted the paragraph to begin and end. I would forget points while writing and couldn't remember what I really wanted to say. I would have to write it down or it would be permanently lost. Then, I struggled to reformat the point in my head. A lot of times my brain would go blank. Thankfully, over the years and with continued treatment for the concussion, pain, and migraines—as well as living a life with lower stress levels—I was able to have fewer blank moments.

When I have a blank moment now, I am able to pull myself through it. It's almost like a moment of anxiety, in a way, but my brain just gets overwhelmed when too much hits it. It's actually not anxiety. It's a neural network injury. Simplistically, when the neuron is trying to deliver its news,[12] it's as if fireworks or a bomb explodes in the neural network. At that point, the brain is overloaded. The brain is in pain. Other parts of the brain are now trying to save the dysfunctioning region of the brain. This is why the healing is slow and people need a controlled environment for healing.

I chose to isolate myself from people. I really wanted a positive atmosphere. I tried to eliminate additional emotional stressors. And, I also controlled my exposure to triggers as much as possible. I recognized my triggers. I stood up for myself. I learned to forgive myself for my errors. I said my weaknesses were now my strengths. I had no weaknesses. This was not because I was arrogant; this was because I was now disabled.

I'm very happy to have moved away from the constant pain, headaches, and migraines. I also now am able to more than likely pull myself through to remember what I was doing. Sometimes I can't. I will just move on to what I am currently doing until I remember what I was doing. However, with continued brain exercise and healing, I hope this will return to normal.

During my pre-accident career, I assisted with developing the Microsoft SharePoint website at Chemical Abstracts Service. I was able to write informational articles, edit coworkers' rough drafts, and analyze material. I was always innovating. I actually couldn't stop innovating. When work was done, I was still innovating. Now, as indicated by my resumes, working took monumental effort. This meant energy. It was frustrating work. It was not enjoyable. It was a chore. I used to be a geek who enjoyed designing graphs. It was my passion. It was like decorating cakes. For others, it was like playing video games. Innovating was a passion. However, as my brain refused to work correctly, I lost passion for writing. No matter how hard I worked, I struggled through infinite pain. The result was always the same. It looked like I was uneducated.

The summer of the accident, I was doing online instruction at Indiana University East. While this was a new position for me, I had lots of experience with teaching. I had taught recitation classes and labs at The Ohio State University as a graduate teaching assistant. I had been head proctor on several occasions. I even had been asked to substitute a review session for the professor one day. I didn't need to provide much supplementary information for my class. The class assignments had already been preloaded for me. All I had to do was show up and teach and grade.

In the fall and spring, I taught in person. I realized I was struggling to find the right words for the pre-lab. During oral instruction, I would struggle to put together a sentence. I couldn't structure it in my head. I couldn't articulate basic algebra or chemistry like I normally could.

I was concerned.

I didn't think it was noticeable to the class, but I could tell. In the past, I could talk about anything with anyone, and I could quickly learn. I even gave a presentation, and the feedback I received was that it was "the most engaging presentation" the group had ever received. Now, here I was teaching, and I was struggling. I was highly concerned.

Years later, I realized that even some of my chemistry knowledge was switched in my head so I really had to focus and jog my memory. For example, my favorite topic in school was backward in my mind. I was adamant I was right until my manager got it into my head. I would like to say a light bulb went off, but it was a real struggle of neuron pathways reconnecting. It was essentially I had the A and B of the pathway, and the neurons were traveling in a jigsaw to get there and crossing each other. The neurons kept hitting the wrong end points until finally something landed.[13] And then I was like, oh yeah, what was I thinking? But that description was exactly how my brain felt. I would explain it as chiseling through a brick wall with a piece of sand. It was painful but muddled. I knew something was happening, but I really wished it would hurry up. Yes, I could actually feel it rewiring. It's energy. And it's not cool. It's really concerning.

I met an HR manager who told me about her struggles with post-concussive syndrome. She said on her bad days, it was like "thinking through rocks and gravel and debris." When she described it, I realized I felt the exact same way. It was literally impossible to think. Now that I've gone

ENERGY, FORCE, AND INTERCONNECTEDNESS

through such a horrible experience (and have finally found a team with a concussion protocol that is working), I have a theory that cognitive fog is a type of pain, perhaps a migraine. Here are some ideas why.

Sadly, a person cannot clean their brain as easily. It's like living in a blurred life and having a moment that clears only a little to connect a thought. However, the thought is still hidden in a fog. Therefore, those with traumatic brain injuries continuously suffer. It takes its toll. It cascades. It doesn't diminish. It worsens and creates more pain and inflammation.

If a medical team can't regulate the inflammation, the post-concussive syndrome worsens. As pain in the brain worsens, the person endures a debilitating life. It may affect other areas of the body as well, because the brain regulates the whole body. It is vital to understand pain in the head, because we have limited resources to resolve worsening issues. A person obviously can't have their head amputated, like a leg amputation, to eliminate inflammation and pain. It is vital to learn about injured neurons and dysfunctioning neuron pathways in order to diagnose and treat brain injuries correctly. Our brains and bodies depend on it.

4.
TAKING LIFE FOR GRANTED

It was really hard to explain what trauma had done. I had taken life for granted—even just doing the little things like in the photos below. I now wondered if these simple movements and positions would ever be possible again. I wondered how much pain I would endure to do these things. They seem so simple. Yet, I could not do them. It took years of hard work to be able to get back into these positions. I still hope to do them like in the pictures someday.

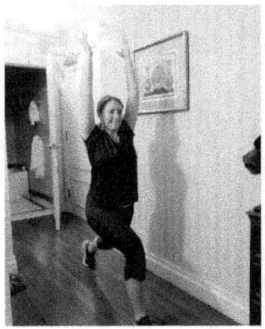
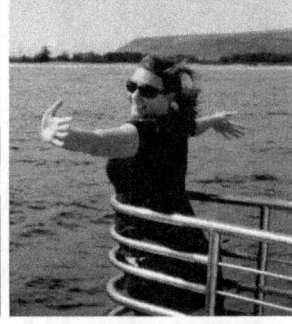

Life actions I took for granted. I could not do these positions after the accident and continue to struggle with them as of 2024.

(From top left) A yoga position from 2016; off the coast of Kauai in 2015; a standing position in Columbus, Ohio; a casual position from 2016.

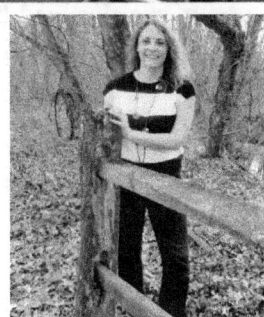
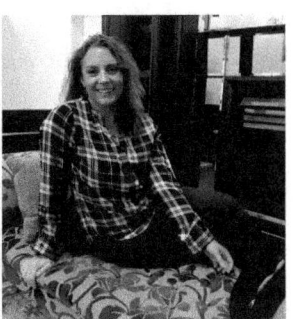

PAIN WITH POISE

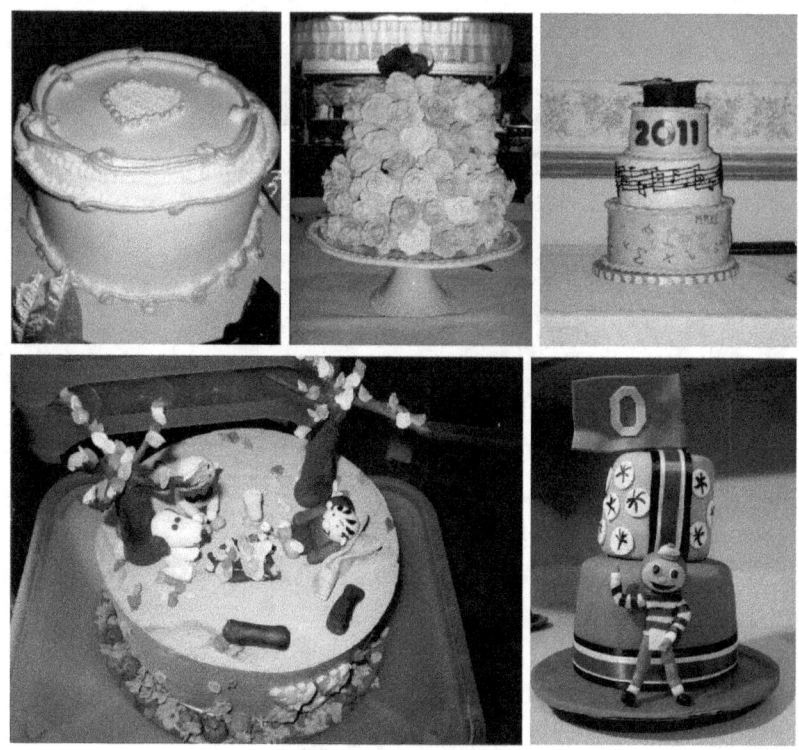

Celebration Cakes I made from 2009-2014.

I continued applying my skills to other hobbies. In 2007, I pursued my passion for baking and decorating cakes. Instead of engineering in the lab, I got to be creative and artistic as a cake designer. I made a *lot* of cakes. I even made my own five-tier wedding cake with gum paste flowers. I learned how to navigate a tiered cake down stairs, over hills, and in traffic.

As a child, I was a terrible athlete. I was unsuccessful in everything: basketball, baseball, tennis, and running. Running hurt. I would always have shin splints. Even walking too much would hurt. This proved true in high school when I joined the volleyball team. I played junior varsity for three years and finally quit. I was never progressing to varsity. While I

TAKING LIFE FOR GRANTED

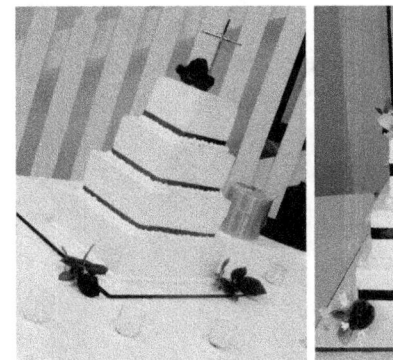
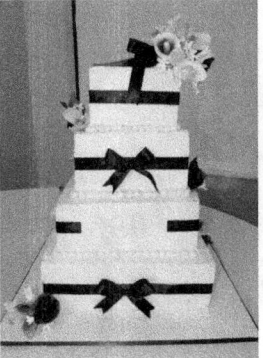
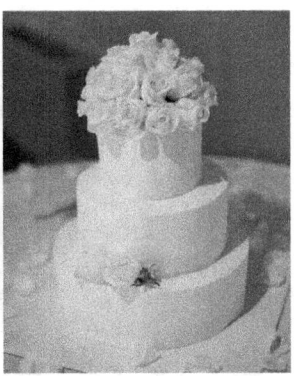

Wedding Cakes from 2009-2014.

could do an overhead serve that impressed everyone, I preferred diving to the floor to save the ball versus running to the ball. I just didn't run.

Then one day in 2010, I met Carey, a retired Marine who encouraged me to start running, and I listened. I signed up for my first 5k and followed the "Couch to 5k" running plan. I then ran my first 5k in the Columbus, Ohio, Capital City Half Marathon in 2011. I fell in love with running, and this began my running journey. I ran several half-marathons over the next few years.

Then, Carey encouraged me to sign up for the Walt Disney World Goofy Challenge in Orlando, Florida. I did sign up. During training, I developed Iliotibial Band Syndrome (ITBS). My sports physician prescribed steroids instead of physical therapy. As I don't like steroids, I didn't take them, and looked online for stretches until post-race. I did cold water soaks after the half marathon, began the full marathon barely able to walk, and finished with ITBS pain. I started and finished the race injured, but I ran 39.3 miles.

I also entered the world of renovating around 2008, when I purchased my first home, a condominium. Since it was a foreclosure, I had to renovate it. For weeks, I went to my job, and then to my condo. I painted, ripped out the old carpet, and put in new floors. I even learned how to cut baseboard. I also began volunteering. I volunteered at several races in the Columbus area, at Lower Lights Ministries in Columbus, Ohio, and at Brookdale Hospice.

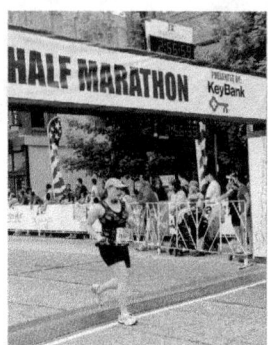 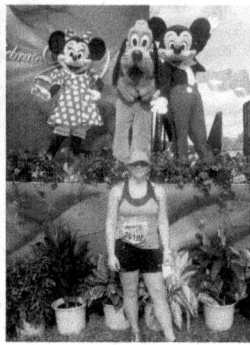 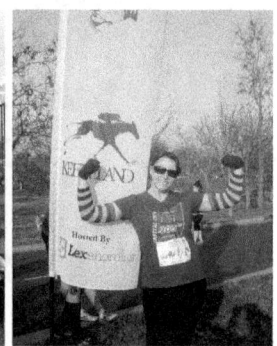

Races from 2012-2013: (Left to right) From 2012 KeyBank The Capital City Half Marathon in Columbus, Ohio; 2013 Walt Disney World Goofy's Race and a Half Challenge in Orlando, Florida; 2013 Run The Bluegrass Half Marathon in Lexington, Kentucky.

5.
THE ALCHEMY OF MY BODY FROM TRAUMA

STRANGER IN CONSCIOUSNESS ALONE

It was a sunny day during the 2020 COVID lockdown when I decided to return to the location my accident had occurred. I had not been there since the day of the accident. I drove for hours following my Garmin GPS. As I got closer to the bank, I suddenly slammed on my brakes.
My Garmin GPS wanted me to turn right at the upcoming intersection. I was on a tiny little two-lane country road. I had stopped beside a two-story white farmhouse and was staring out across acres and acres of farmland. I saw a stop sign to my right. The main road was just feet away. It appeared unfamiliar but, I just knew somehow inside of me that this was the location of my accident.

I crept to the stop sign. I stopped and looked. I saw the large road that went for miles and miles just feet across from me. If I crossed the main road, I would be on it. Instead, I sat and stared at the green farmland and wondered. How did my brain and body recognize the location from the wrong direction? I was troubled.

I turned right. I continued my drive to the bank, but I was shocked to drive through a town. The town had a red light. I had no memory of this town. Nothing made sense. Then, I made it to the bank. I recognized the bank and the area around the bank.

But, in my head, the accident happened as soon as I pulled out from the bank parking lot. The farmland had just appeared after the bank parking lot in my head. I sat at the bank and then began driving the fateful route home.

As I drove, I exited the town and immediately started hysterical sobbing. I kept driving while I sobbed. I had no idea where I was or where I was going until the hysterical sobs were over. When the sobs stopped, I realized I had passed the accident scene, the house, and had arrived at the interstate.

My body and nerves knew the accident scene. My consciousness did not. That's when I started to get really concerned about what was wrong with my brain that we didn't know about yet.

Essentially, the hysterical sobbing is my body showing signs of distress and how it went through sheer terror the day of the accident. On other attempts to return to the accident site, I fail because my brain starts driving me in circles until I am forced to give up and return home.

TRAUMA MEMORY

When the body is attacked, the brain moves into action to save it. This is the case whether a person is conscious or unconscious. In the case of an impact event, there is an impact connection with the brain to those nerves in the region of the body affected by the impact. The affected nerves send pain information to the brain, which interprets the pain information.

Even unconscious and unaware, the brain is awake and functioning to save a person's life. It hears things, feels things, and smells things that the conscious self may not remember. These unconscious memories become a part of the person. These realities become both unconscious and subconscious memories that the person may never consciously realize.

To discuss trauma memory, one has to understand a memory. We all have memories from experience in real time that are associated with another person, both positive or negative. This is why I believe a memory of a bad event is not always trauma. What makes a memory a trauma memory requires a combination of things. There has to be something in that bad event that triggers something within a person to qualify it as a trauma memory.

It has to cross a trauma threshold. This trauma threshold is different for everyone. Perhaps, some people have better coping mechanisms so when something bad happens it doesn't cause a trauma memory. Maybe that particular bad event was something that literally didn't matter to a person, therefore it never formed a trauma memory in that person.

I came to this theory after evaluating several traumatic events in my life—including the tractor-trailer accident—and how I handled them.

A GREAT BETRAYAL

The first traumatic event I evaluated occurred in 2013. I had always been reticent about chiropractors, but I decided to try one to heal a stubborn running injury. It worked, but the chiropractor caressed my knee at my last visit. It was extremely horrifying. By the time I figured out what was happening, I had decided to shove my foot in his face. Then, he quit caressing my knee and got out of the way. Remembering what police officers had always said in rape defense training growing up, I had stared the man down. When I went to leave the room, the chiropractor followed me. Not to be beaten, I turned around to meet him, and he wanted to shake my hand. I gave it to him and snarled at him. It was the first time in my life I had ever hated a person. Then, I went to my car and cried knowing my old life was over. My precious, innocent, happy life just ended. I had encountered a predator.

I told my then husband. I told my running buddy. I told my best friend. I told my parents. I told a lot of people. I told coworkers who were really concerned for me. I told my counselor. I reported it to the police and learned it was not a crime. I told my gynecologist and my family doctor. I had everybody covered. And I had a life to live, so I moved forward. The memory only crept into my mind once every few months, if that. It was over.

PAIN WITH POISE

In 2015, my marriage to a police officer ended. After my divorce with my ex, I went to Kauai to visit family and celebrated with my friend Jennifer. I was doing what made me happy. I took charge. I was in no pain. Whatever my ex-husband had said, I left behind. Then, I came home. I was ghosted and unfriended by very close friends—because of the divorce. Yet, I still had my church.

Then, people from church began interfering. They had all these rules for me. Some weren't even married and they were giving me rules. They were telling me I had to wait a year to date. I was not getting invited to events. They uninvited me to birthday parties. I was shocked. I was a minister's daughter who had endured just about everything in a church, including church splits caused by church politics. Yet, I had never been spiritually abused or shunned by a church. To worsen matters, an individual from the church attempted to control me with an unnecessary wellness check. This could even be classified as a swatting event. It was extremely disturbing.

While all events left a scar memory in my brain, not all of the traumatic events left me with the same long-lasting trauma. As I had little stress from the knee caress trauma and getting divorced, I did not suffer from trauma. I knew not having a man was not the end of my world. During the possible swatting event, I learned my "no" didn't matter. My voice had been silenced. I no longer felt comfortable in my house, on my property, in my car, in a church, or around cops. I did develop trauma. As it happened by church people, it really harmed me. I felt unsafe and powerless. I grieved the loss of my voice, my freedom, power, and pride. This time I developed trauma.

Because these traumas continued for years, I was unable to find a reprieve. I stayed stressed from the constant disruptions. I lost some of my confidence. I began rethinking who I was and what I was to be in life. This domino effect led me to think God had turned his back on me to make me endure a new spiritual journey. I kept quoting, "Eli, Eli, lama sabachthani."

Interpreted, this means, "My God, My God, why have You forsaken Me?"[1] The trials in my life had reached such an overwhelming and odd extreme that it felt like "hell on Earth." I could still tell myself no matter how insurmountable the challenges and shocking my life had become, I continued striving forward knowing it was not because of me that this was happening. Jesus had been perfect when he had been crucified.

NERVES—AND THE ALTERED AWARENESS

However, I encountered a major issue when recovering from the 18-wheeler accident. The injury was severe, and I was living in debilitating pain. I was exercising and soon realized my pain was increasing. I began to experience more trauma as my pain increased. I didn't want to experience the pain. Therefore, my physical therapy sessions suffered. It made me wonder if there was a direct link between pain and trauma. I already had some trauma leaving the hospital, but the trauma worsened as I exercised.

As I worked different muscles, I would relive the accident. While I had been knocked unconscious and had no memory of any impact, my brain had still been working, resulting in memories to be stored in my unconscious and subconscious mind. These memories were of what my brain did to keep me alive, what my body reflexively did, and all the sensory information to which the nerves were exposed.

As I performed certain movements in life, the trauma would hit. As we worked certain muscles in physical therapy, the subconscious memory would sometimes reach my conscious memory. While it was not known to my conscious memory as being a real memory of the accident—for the simple reason I had been unconscious—my body still recognized it. My subconscious was now one with my conscious. It was a trauma memory. The problem with becoming one with a trauma memory was the sickness that ensued.

My trauma memory journey began by being mostly fascinated and curious about semi-trailer trucks. I began to be curious about the position

PAIN WITH POISE

of my head in relation to the tires of a semi-truck and my head placement on the metal rim. I studied the 18-wheeler one day and realized my head gash was level with the bottom rim of the trailer. Then, I was in awe of the size of the tire of an 18-wheeler. I wanted to know the ins and outs of what happened to me. I wanted to know the science. I wanted to understand the miracle. I wanted to learn.

It felt like I was living in shock for months and even years after being hit by the semi-trailer truck. I lived and moved through the world like I wasn't fully there. In the beginning, I would sit at home and just say, "I was hit by a tractor-trailer." Then, I would laugh like a hyena. During this phase, I would tell anybody who would listen that I was hit by a semi-trailer. It was as if I were discussing my passions. Then, I went through a phase where I would just randomly text people "I was hit by a tractor-trailer."

When this phase ended, I could no longer say I had been hit by an 18-wheeler, because it brought about deep ugly pain, extreme soul-wrenching sadness, and a brick to my brain. What I once was able to speak of freely was now deeply entrenched like a scar tissue. It had healed in gnarly, nasty memories that changed me completely. The only reason I laughed like a hyena was because I was not able to process what had truly happened to me yet. Quite frankly, those around me should have been very scared of me when I laughed like a hyena.

Sometimes, I had superhuman strength. The causes were debatable. Were the surges due to adrenaline from trauma? Was it due to high levels of pain? Was it thinking I had defeated a semi-trailer? Was it a combination of both? Other times, I would be a superhuman who was untouchable. Was it because I had met God? Was it because I had met the devil? Was it that I had overcome things that other humans had not? Was it because I now looked at things from a godly wisdom and not from a worldly wisdom? Was it because I now viewed things in a drastically different way than other humans, and this extreme clash made me think humans were really stupid?

THE ALCHEMY OF MY BODY FROM TRAUMA

In the beginning, the only way I could describe very good days was walking forward with my normal, exuberant personality while my left side wanted to falter and shy away and hide. I would fight the desire to fall back into my shell of protection, which was like another personality. As I had been knocked unconscious, I will never know if my body touched any part of the 18-wheeler directly. However, the left side of my body saw it and had sustained the maximum energy, if not at minimum, indirect impact, while my right side never saw it. The semi-trailer truck did not want me to have a life of exuberance, carefree lightheartedness, and happiness. I was to be negative, mean, and crude. The semi-truck was a monster. I slowly evolved into a zombie. I felt like I was both dead and living. I felt nothing like a human.

One day in 2018, I found my storage of childhood stuffed animals. Through the years, my mom had sent them to me when she was cleaning their house, and I just stored them in a closet. I picked up one of my largest stuffed animals and held it for a little bit. Then, I set it back in the closet. When I started to pull my hands away, I was shocked to see my hands and arms violently shaking. The movement was very violent as it was tight and constricted. I felt no anxiety in my body. I felt no breathing change. It was just my arms and hands.

I decided it was a sign I needed my teddy bear. I felt weird. I was an adult and I was sleeping with a stuffed animal. But, I had also been through a truly horrific accident. I learned how few people had been hit by tractor-trailers.

I was going to sleep with my teddy bear.

After about a year, I decided to try a body pillow to substitute the teddy bear. They were the same size. I could let go of the teddy bear and not have the same response, but I don't know if it really worked. Teddy bears still protect a person in a special way.

I would go through a phase of blowing kisses at semi-trailer trucks. However, that was not out of victory or cockiness, but instead trauma. I

PAIN WITH POISE

think that was more from how close my lips were to touching the 18-wheeler. I believe my brain interpreted the sensation as a kiss. Then, I would have times when turning left made me see a semi-trailer truck coming at me.

Very soon after the accident, a trauma episode occurred when a song came on over the speaker at Kohl's, and I envisioned dancing with a tractor-trailer. This was when I started thinking that I don't even know what song was playing on the radio when I was hit. I don't know the beat of the song at impact. This means I don't know the beat or song or singer or band that will trigger my trauma.

Then, I would go through phases of having sensations of things hitting my face and my chin. To make sense of them, I had the urge to slam my chin into the coffee table. I fought this urge several nights. Sometimes, my back would ripple like ball bats were beating it. With each impact, I would want to physically act out the ripples. When things like that happened, I didn't know what came first: the spasms or the trauma. They were both related. Was it the trauma that came with the spasms or the spasms that came with the trauma? However, once my back healed to a certain level, the sensations of it being beat disappeared.

I described trauma as having a split brain. This split brain was not the medical split brain, where the corpus callosum of the brain is removed.[2] Instead, trauma split brain is when two worlds live in the brain simultaneously. I lived in the world of the accident and the current world together. Since there was so much nerve memory involved in trauma, maybe split body was appropriate to describe the trauma as well. It's not just a memory. It is a whole-body experience.

I would do my job serving customers and talking to customers while fighting waves of ball bats and ripples to my back. I would clean while having blurred gray objects swirling through my mind's vision. The most exhausting part of my day was trying to block the trauma so I could be a functional human. Who wants to feel baseball bats beating a back at random times during the day?

THE ALCHEMY OF MY BODY FROM TRAUMA

In 2019, I almost suffocated because I had long hair. I was going through a phase of trauma where I needed my hair gone immediately. I made an appointment and told my hairdresser the truth. "I'm going to suffocate. Cut it off." She cut it the shortest it had been since high school. It was below the chin. The length worked. I stopped having the trauma episodes.

In 2021, I found a news article with a picture of the accident I had never seen before. I started crying an inhuman cry. With the cry came an uncontrollable leaning to my right, and rolling my left shoulder forward. I just kept leaning. Only after it stopped was I able to think about the strange behavior. I only later realized the picture had triggered trauma. I can only surmise it was my body re-enacting the motions during the semi-trailer truck impact the day of the accident.

I developed several coping mechanisms. I tried texting people through the trauma. It was hard talking to people through the trauma. One night, I lay on my stomach enduring the spasms and trauma while texting my buddy Randy. I would feel the impact in my back, and shimmers raced across it. I could only imagine it was what my back and nerves imprinted when the 18-wheeler impacted it.

I compared it to watching a movie in the cinema and seeing the percussion waves during a fighting scene impacting my back. I needed friends who could respond immediately. Another coping mechanism was going to the grocery late at night when it was still 24/7 pre-COVID. This also gave me a safer location to be at night since sometimes I felt claustrophobic.

In 2021, I had a moment where I felt drilled through the left side of my head to the center. The sensation was not painful. I once endured the sensation of being skinned along my left side: along my jaw and cheek and eye. It felt like a razor was being taken to it. Still another time, I woke up and it felt like I was hit by a car. I jumped out of bed. All the nerves in my body were alive, including my arms, hands, spine, and head, and it felt like I had been impacted hard. These were the times I was left wondering who I was and what I might become…and if I would ever return to normal.

PAIN WITH POISE

In 2023, I began experiencing something new. The left side of my face would spasm so intensely that I would sob. It felt like it was being rearranged. While I had experienced far worse pain through this ordeal, there is nothing like having one's body be rearranged. I might compare it to a person having a dislocated shoulder. It was like having something living in my face; like I had a snake slithering through my face. Saliva would gather in my mouth. I would cry violently. I would always have to spit the pooled saliva out. Eventually, I realized my saliva was often mixed with blood. This seemed linked to my persistent facial issues. Eventually the blood disappeared.

After one particularly bad episode, my head felt alive with nerves. I couldn't sleep. Finally, I got out of bed and immediately my brain began to feel like it was vibrating violently in my skull. I screamed a high-pitched, shrill scream. The pain was unimaginable. It was indescribable. Then, it was over. My brain was normal, and I was relaxed and went to sleep. The nerve sensations I had been feeling where my head felt alive vanished. I woke up the next morning. I had an MRI, and it was normal. Maybe it was energy. Maybe it was a spasm. Maybe something was healing.

IDENTITY CRISIS—SUFFOCATED BY GRIEF

As I went through my recovery, the chronic pain changed me. People were so quick to talk about the emotional trauma and psychological trauma of events that they would forget that physical trauma existed as well. Chronic pain, combined with the emotional and psychological trauma I experienced, changed me forever. The extreme experience, extreme effort put into recovery, and the traumatic brain injury all added up.

On top of this, I began to deal with grief. With each step backward in physical therapy, I started to grieve. With each encounter with a difficult medical team, I grieved more. With each loss of a job, I grieved more. With each day I was still at a job not financially aligned with my goals,

THE ALCHEMY OF MY BODY FROM TRAUMA

I grieved. With each struggle to lose weight, I grieved. With each struggle to get my day to return to a habit, I grieved. Every day my original goals grew further away or were achieved with insurmountable effort, I grieved. Every time my family struggled, I grieved. As the grief increased, my trauma increased.

I used to be so organized and everything came so easily to me. I had a strong body with a healthy, strong brain. I could keep my house and organize my day. Now, everything was injured. Every day I had to go to another medical appointment. It was another day lost to sickness.

Post-accident, I began to experience a personality change. I had a concussion complicated by trauma, long-term extreme pain, frustrating physical rehabilitation, and difficult medical interactions with staff and doctors. Some of those interactions might even be considered abusive. I also endured so much stress from physical rehabilitation and financial obligations that I became a different person. There was a person who remembered the old me, because she lived in that person's house, saw her in pictures, and wore that person's clothes. Yet, that person was not who I had become.

A lot of things contributed to this personality change. I was under an extreme amount of stress. I endured medical teams that were not very professional and caused me significant distress. My goal to keep my stress low backfired, and it was because I couldn't live in a bubble. I had to do research to try and find a medical team that might heal me more efficiently. I was still juggling jobs. In the end, the lack of rest and all the stressors drained my positive energy. I didn't have any free time.

Stress could trigger more than just trauma. It could exacerbate a person's post-concussive syndrome, neuromuscular conditions, cardiovascular conditions, and even increase pain levels. There was a reason I had always tried to manage the stress in my life. I was a low-key person, and while I liked a full life, I planned well with few disruptions to have a very stress-free life. There were positive disruptions and negative disruptions. There were innovative disruptions and catastrophic disruptions.

PAIN WITH POISE

I believed in managing stress so it did not control me. I really liked to just let things go and walk away and disengage. This was one of the main reasons I was so angry at my medical team for not listening to me when I said I was in pain, and not taking me seriously about it being too early to return to work.

It was also why jumping through hoops to get the appropriate ADA paperwork for work was so infuriating. These were needless disruptions. They were catastrophic. They were unhealthy. They were not innovative disruptions. Life was full of these stressful disruptions, causing me more and more inflammation, which was increasing my pain.

I expected to suffer from physical pain and even trauma. I had not expected to suffer at the extreme rate I did from pain due to the lack of effective medical treatment, additional navigating to find proper treatment, and anxiety from being abused by medical staff. I was enduring psychological and emotional stress unrelated to trauma. I was now facing cultural suffering as I was in a new world where my disability resulted in a lack of inclusion and new professional struggles. I also faced problems as I was a woman with a disability. I was ignored.

I was suffering financial pains like other sick, disabled people, or those living in pain. I was economically suffering from my dire finances and owing more in medical bills. I was also facing additional economical pains the entire time I was trying to heal, as I was not able to get a job to cover my bills. Previously, I had been accustomed to a job with plenty of disposable income.

As I went along this journey, my identity crisis was real. I no longer responded to or liked the name Ashley. I did not know who Ashley was. I told people that was my name, but I really wanted to go by another one. Ashley was so foreign to me. Ashley belonged to another person. My grandmother had a problem with her name when she grew up and had changed its spelling. I really thought about changing my legal name. In the pronoun world, I still associated as a she/her, but I think that was only because of my very religious upbringing. I think I could have gone with "it" or "they" because I didn't feel like anything. I didn't feel human.

The name didn't make my heart sing. It didn't make me feel beautiful. It didn't resonate with me. Ashley was not me. Maybe I still don't resonate with Ashley. Sometimes, the name is still all wrong. Yet, it's my name. As the years have passed, Aunt Ashley has now become my favorite name.

SPIRITUAL ENLIGHTENMENT

As the daughter of a retired Baptist minister, I was used to God. As a child, I went to church, participated in church activities, and sang in choir. I taught classes, in both scripture and music, to kids of all ages at church. I never got into trouble. I was a great church kid. However, I was really burnt out of the church thing when I moved to Columbus, Ohio.

Shortly after moving to Columbus in 2004, I began questioning my religion. I was meeting so many people and was challenged in so many new ways that I was having new questions. I looked at my grandpa, a minister of southern Ohio, and asked him about it. He said, "Ashley, we may have everything wrong about the Bible, because we (humans) are interpreting it. What matters is that we get to heaven."

My grandpa made me really stop and think. My whole life I thought my religion had been right. Now, my grandpa was telling me we could be wrong. It was thought-provoking. I did firmly believe I had become a Christian in 1991. While I do believe Jesus is the way to heaven, I couldn't verify that Baptists had come up with the magic process to get to heaven. I became more cautious in my religion. I questioned more. I still held onto God, though.

As I formed answers to my questions, I deepened my religious philosophy. I decided I didn't like the idea of divided religion, and that this prevented everyone from being able to focus on one true goal: God. I still strongly held on to my core beliefs, but I began looking at religion from another perspective. In 2014, I began a new relationship with God.

I realized I could tell God anything, in any manner, and God would love me. It was mostly the realization that God already knew me thoroughly, because he already had access to my brain. For this reason, I decided it was silly to filter any bad thoughts or angry thoughts from God. I also praised God abundantly and learned to know and love a new God. This radical transparency mattered a lot with my relationship with God when I began the tractor-trailer recovery. God got all my hate, confusion, and anger.

I thought back to before the semi-truck accident, when I had been saying, "Eli, Eli, lama sabachthani."[3] During those trials, I thought I had gone through hell. But now, I was praising God for saving my life in a miraculous way. In fact, I met God the day the semi-trailer truck hit me. He did not turn his back on me that day. He flew to me. The grace and mercy I experienced in all of God's awe that day made me appreciate the greatness of my God. The advice from churches and ministers was no longer useful. I was interpreting everything differently. I was on a new journey with God.

I began deep philosophical thinking about God, life, and death after the accident. Since God had allowed my eyes to open, I had to face a long recovery. During this time, I both praised God, hated God, and yelled at God. God could've let my eyes remain closed. If God had chosen death for me, then I would never have known pain. I would have been in perfect happiness and in peace. Since he didn't let my eyes remain closed, I began a journey of spiritual turmoil.

Since I was not with God in heaven, I believed I had failed him. Even with the old reminder that I was God's princess, it was not enough in the darkest of the dark to keep me from reaching my own Job.[4] My sorrow was real. I also struggled with survivor's guilt. I was alive while so many people died from tractor-trailer motor vehicle accidents. Why was I so lucky instead of them? Would people hate me because I was alive? Was I allowed to be honest about how I felt? I began a journey of guilt, anger, joy, and hate. I lived under a shadow of shame.

For months after the accident, I heard sounds in my head. They varied in volume from loud screams to a soft voice. The voice was a simple phrase that puzzled me. It said, simply, "I love you, mommy and daddy." I thought on those words for a while. Could they have been my last words thinking I was going to die? Were they my last thoughts? What happened that I do not remember? I pondered on these thoughts along with the sights of the being made of a flame and in a robe.

While grappling with death one day in 2018, I got in my car and drove 45 minutes to Dayton. I drove until I saw a tower in the distance and kept taking turn after turn as if guided by a mysterious force. Then, I saw a tiny country church with a cemetery. I drove through the cemetery to the back of it. At the back was a little pond as well as the oldest tombstones. There were not many tombstones, and it was a very pretty farmland area. Then, I did the strangest thing. I found a little grassy patch and lay down beside the tombstones. I was tired of dealing with real life, because it didn't make sense. Death and dead people made sense to me. In that moment, I felt at home.

That night, while I lay in my bed to sleep, I felt like I was one of the dead. I felt like I was decaying with bugs crawling on me, but not in a creepy way. I felt like I was surrounded by men in Civil War uniforms. Instead of telling myself it was my wild imagination, I said it was my new connections to those in the afterlife sharing their views. I firmly believed their energies were being shared. They had a story to tell. There was a reason I was led there silently that day. Those people were no longer in pain.

As I continued to think about death, I recalled how my grandpa, Ted, stated each year after he had retired, "This is the year I will die." My grandpa was not a depressed man. He was quite the opposite. He lived a joyous and full life. He was a minister and he really loved his God. He was just eager to meet his God. As the years passed, years came and went and he did not die. Then one year, decades later, he finally did pass away. One year, his statement became true.

This only aided in my new understanding of death and life. There

PAIN WITH POISE

was nothing wrong with saying or even expecting to die. Death was natural. I learned to accept this truth after the tractor-trailer hit me. One day, we all die. While I had always known everybody would die, I now intimately knew death. I had faced death. God had let me beat death. Now, the question became: Was this a blessing or a curse?

As I was alive, I was living in pain and dealing with an uphill battle of managing finances, pain management, healing my body, and maintaining social connections. I was navigating hearings and legal battles. I was in a world that no longer resembled my life. I could not fathom why God had let me "open my eyes." I'd had a chance at achieving real peace in heaven and leaving this planet.

Strangely, I then developed a new fear. Where I had once been young and fearless, I now feared death. I had tasted it. The next time I faced death, I would now face pain. A heart attack would not be a peaceful death. Dying of cancer would not be a peaceful death. I was mad God had let my eyes reopen. For me, dying from the 18-wheeler would have been painless.

Because of the pain I experienced after the accident, the lack of support, and the many struggles, I decided God hated me. My doctors were not helping me. I was starting to think my injury was really severe, and I would be disabled forever. I had originally thought it would be a quick fix. People who had been in my very situation were dead. Why was I alive and required to endure it? I couldn't figure out why God would want me to suffer so much.

I decided God hated me and I was a really bad person. I became very angry at God. Everything I had done in life must have been bad and it had angered God. Somehow, he was very angry with me, because I was not dead. God had to hate me to make me endure this horrendous suffering.

As the years went by, I also got angry at God because I was supposed to be this tough. To be this tough and to endure this hell was a curse. I

THE ALCHEMY OF MY BODY FROM TRAUMA

didn't want to be tough. I began hating myself and my toughness. And the tests to show how tough I was were piling up. Why could I not have family and friends in my house like everyone else? I wanted to be laughing with them. I didn't want to be texting with them. I was starting to face the horror that my injury was really severe and I would be disabled forever.

Why could I not be that woman whose biggest struggle was a fight with her husband or a flat tire? Or the woman whose biggest struggle in life was her homeowner's association not liking the color of her roof? For the first time in my life, I stooped to a new level. I actually used the "it's not fair" phrase. I had always prided myself on not going there. But the challenges were ripping me to shreds.

I still tried to read my Bible. I established the daily goal of one Bible verse a day. This lasted a bit. Then, I would just open my Bible and read whatever passage I would open to, like I used to do. I always considered it God-inspired or God directing me to a passage. I was reading the Bible and I began to notice a problem. Over the years, my Bible reading evolved to hearing constant criticisms of myself. Out of all my time as a Christian, I've never had an issue like this, not even under conviction. I finally said: This is not of God. God doesn't belittle. He doesn't point out our faults.

The Bible was angering me. I became so frustrated that I could not read it the way I used to that I began throwing my Bible. I became enraged. It was like all I heard was the devil when I read the Bible instead of God. It was like it had become the devil's Bible.

God reminded me that Moses broke the tablets inscribed with the 10 Commandments,[5] so I felt okay that I threw my Bible. Humans can't handle close encounters with God. For example, Moses glowed from encountering God at the burning bush.[6] God changed people. Experiencing God was too much for me after the accident.

Connecting with God when reading my Bible simply became too emotionally overwhelming for me. For lack of a better explanation, it was like being overtaken by an explosion of energy when knowing God. To know a God who could understand all the extremes I was experiencing as I began to understand God more and more with each experience was formidable. I simultaneously experienced immense suffering and indescribable, overflowing joy for being graced with a rare, precious gift: LIFE.

While I attempted to unravel these searing, conflicting emotions, I knew one thing. God already knew every emotion I was feeling. God didn't stress me. He just knew. I was really glad I didn't have to put myself through more pain to pray to God based on church rules. He didn't judge me like humans. God was really accepting and it was easy to tell him the truth.

God also knew what I was enduring even better than I did—which was even more awe-inspiring and love-inducing and overpowering than I could handle. That overwhelmed me with gratefulness. God was so much bigger than the Bible. When I held my Bible in my hands, it was too small. God was bigger than the Universe. He cannot be restricted to a Bible. The Bible did not save me from death. God did.

I struggled when I realized how much control God really had. I had a misunderstanding of what control was before this tractor-trailer journey. The control I knew of was a mirage. It would be like watching a magician perform a magical act. I walked from a vehicle where I was saved only by God. Satan did not save me that day, but he did his best to end my life. God and my angels fought Satan for me. Spiritual warfare is where miracles happen. God knew every cell that Satan injured that day. I began a long, long new journey fighting Satan. It may not have felt like it at times, but God loved me.

Knowing how much control God has does not make me feel safe. In fact, I feel bare and naked. I am reminded of Jesus and the cross. Jesus didn't want to die on the cross. Yet, he knew God was in control. God could have saved Jesus so that Jesus never had to die for us. However, God loved us and chose Jesus as a sacrifice to forgive all our sins. Jesus, in fact, was under so much stress that his sweat resembled blood.[7] That is a lot of stress.

THE ALCHEMY OF MY BODY FROM TRAUMA

Now, by being hit by a semi-truck, I feel like I know Jesus a whole lot more, and I respect the control that God has a lot more even if it's terrifying. I also know God could ask me to do things that make me completely unhappy. God does not ask us to do things that make us happy. Some things that God asks us to do are counter-intuitive and horrible, like dying on a cross or staying alive while in horrible pain. Spiritual enlightenment is rough.

6.
THE SLAP

Counterintuitive to my healing, I began a practice of slapping myself. My face was on fire, contorting, and I was stuck in a pain hell. The slaps were fresh and new. Since I was weak at first, the slaps barely stung. However, I was still slapping myself and I noticed my skin was bleeding; it looked like it was falling off. Still, slapping became a part of my life. I used slaps for so many different reasons.

My pain was so searing that a slap helped ease the pain. It was like using fire to take out a fire. My face burned. It was only an instinct, or animal reaction. It was not anything I had read about until I was researching for my own book. This is when I learned that people who suffer from migraines will create other sources of pain to distract from the pain of the headache, such as pulling out their hair. I was in total misery.

When I was put on my nerve pain medications, I noticed something. After a few weeks of being on my nerve medications, even with the continued slaps, I stopped having issues with my skin. Even off the medications today, I still slap myself. Today the slap is a harder slap, because I have more strength than I did after the accident. Unfortunately, these may include the added strength of a muscle spasm. But, my skin doesn't bleed or try to fall off. It reacts just like it did pre-accident. I think this is an important observation. I believe I was suffering from nerve irritability that was affecting my skin's health due to the accident. Therefore, a slap caused me to easily bleed and lose skin. With the nerve pain medication, it allowed my nerves to heal enough to let my skin heal.

PAIN WITH POISE

Grief became the new norm in my life. When grief became overwhelming, I slapped myself. Other times, it was because people bossed me around or thought they knew better than me. This brought about more grief and confusion. I couldn't explain myself. I couldn't find the words. It could even be their tone. I was no longer able to process tones.

I was doing jobs that were under my education and experience level. It was really hard on my ego. Other times, people were offering sabotage advice. These people meant well, but they were really sabotaging my future and options. The tractor-trailer wasn't going to take my goals. It just changed the journey. I slapped myself when people tried to redirect me so I could stay on *their* right path.

In addition, my physical pain levels were so high I was losing my filter. I would try to not say the wrong things, but that would rev my physical pain up to explosion levels. I would have to slap myself. The slap became an exothermic reaction for me. I could no longer contain the energy that was trying to be released via pain, words, screams, and more. I slapped everything back inside. Losing my filter was the release of the monster I didn't even want to meet. It had to go back in its cage. I had to be that savvy analyst go-getter again.

Slaps don't harm people when a person does it to themselves. A slap was equal to screaming and crying. A slap was trying to come alive again. A slap was trying to feel human. My slaps were not going to bother anyone either. Later, I saw on TV where a woman who endured great trauma shared that she slapped herself. If a woman who endured great trauma slaps herself, then I could slap myself from trauma or pain. I was hit by a semi-trailer truck. I live for the day I don't slap myself anymore, but until then, it means I am alive.

7.
SANITY IN AN INSANE WORLD

As I continued along the process of my recovery with the weeks turning into months, I began to learn my new body. Part of the misery of life after the accident was reliving trauma that my body and nerves remembered, but my conscious did not. It was during this time that I legitimately felt like a monster.

The 18-wheeler energies were now part of me, causing malfunctions, and releasing my monster. I was a mess, and I could not stop it. If people judged me or didn't support me, I realized they were lacking in the knowledge that I had once lacked. Trauma was a horror that was unable to be explained. To make it worse, trauma was interlaced and inseparable from pain.

During my recovery, someone asked me if I had ever experienced pain that was comparable to that of stage 4 cancer. I could not answer. I didn't know what stage 4 cancer pain felt like. I also didn't know what it felt like to be burned alive and then have to lie in a hospital bed to have sheets ripped off a bleeding and raw back. Was my pain equivalent to either of those horrific scenarios? I didn't know. I had not had either experience.

What I had experienced was pain from impact energies from a tractor-trailer traveling 50 mph. A person with stage 4 cancer cannot tell me her pain was worse than my semi-trailer truck pain. It was impossible for a stage 4 cancer patient to know my pain without being hit by a tractor-trailer themselves. I was faced with a quandary. I didn't know how to describe my pain. It was insanity to tell me my pain was less than somebody else to subdue me or put me in place.

PAIN WITH POISE

Another perspective regarding pain was from my time as a runner. When I averaged running 40 miles to finish the 2013 Goofy Challenge, I ached a lot. I hobbled. That was a 2/10 on the pain scale compared to being hit by a tractor-trailer.

To cope with this soreness, marathoners walk backward, take the stairs backward, and all this crazy stuff after a marathon because of sore muscles. Marathoners even continue running during a marathon, because it hurts less to transition from walking to running. That soreness was not how I felt after a semi-trailer truck hit me. This is why being hit by an 18-wheeler changed my perspective on pain.

As I added back my daily activities and tried to have a career, I started screaming internally for morphine. I would tell people I thought I needed morphine. I was barely functioning. I woke in agonizing pain, and my pain only worsened through the day. I could no longer cope with the pain. I was rubbing the inside of my hands with my fingers until they bruised. I would fidget with my arms or wrists. I started screaming these alarming, high-pitched screams that didn't even seem to come from me.

I was no longer able to cry. My head felt like molten lava. My eyes felt like quicksand. I felt pieced together, part by part, and nothing worked together. Each piece was put together incorrectly and belonged to another person. I felt like Frankenstein's monster.

As my body did more and more crazy things over time from the damage it had sustained, reality slowly sank in. Then, came the real horror. I couldn't look away. I couldn't wake up and have the nightmare be over. I couldn't change the channel to get away. My pain, my trauma, and fighting to overcome them was now my life, and I had to stay with it. With this realization, I changed. I couldn't stay the same. I started slapping myself to endure and keep going.

With this change came a new issue—I could no longer handle other people's traumas. I was trauma'd out. For example, I avoided everything about remembering 9/11 for years. I switched the channel on everything that had to do with the suffering of people in other countries. I could no longer watch the news. I could handle nothing about crime.

Even when the Russo-Ukraine War started in 2022, I was only able to take it in initially before quickly burning out. When COVID-19 came around, I really did not care. Nobody was allowed to even mention the semi-truck to me. That was too much trauma. It had nothing to do with me being out of touch with reality. It was quite the opposite.

I was now carrying burdens that made me look at the world differently; the sane living in an insane world. The world around me was making insane decisions. Bureaucracy was futile in dealing with the reality of the cruelties of this world. I behaved differently. I was under extreme pressure from instant change, which resulted in strange behaviors and weirdness. I needed to learn who I was supposed to become and what my new world would be.

I was a person with trauma. That made me a warrior. As a warrior, I was still fighting long after the event was over. When people suffering from trauma reach out to another person, they can't be ignored, abused, or considered a mental mess. They are going through a really tough time unlike anything others will ever know. I compare it to an Alcoholics Anonymous group. If a recovering alcoholic is at the bar and they need to call their AA sponsor, they need to know their sponsor will be there. Guess what? They need humans who are there for them and respect them. This is the same for people with trauma. People with trauma are misunderstood.

Of course, I could use a counselor to help me determine my new self, yet, how many counselors had been hit by 18-wheelers? I considered it dangerous to even talk to one. Counselors were not God. They did not know the future God had in store for me. The sane reality was I had been hit by a tractor-trailer. The world expected insanity for me to blend. In reality, it was no different than a perfect Jesus coming to earth to walk on a sinful earth.

It was amazing what humans needed me to do to re-conform to society. I had to go to a job. I had to work a predetermined shift. I needed detailed descriptions of what I could and could not do filled out on a piece of paper. I had to fill out a calendar of appointments. Peer pressure from websites and commercials showed the latest technology for reducing toxins, restoring fascia health, and providing miracle cures. Diets and vitamins were suggested by friends and medical providers to alleviate trauma, concussions, and overall health. Most were not even proven. The life I was supposed to blend into was insanity. Everyone had the miracle cure, the answer. Order, structure, rules. Everyone was eager and expected things to return to a normal life.

Yet, I had endured the supernatural. My own genes had been modified.[1] The tractor-trailer energy had become me. From a biological and metaphysical standpoint, Ashley was no longer. She was new. It was a rebirth. I just wanted to live my new life. Was I sane because of my trauma reality? Was I sane because I was now one with the Universe and not humans? Was I sane because I walked with God? I did not know. I just knew I no longer knew the world and it had become foreign to me. I could not conform because it hurt me. I just wanted to experience the beauty of it. And so, I began experiencing everything anew.

8.
LIFE AND RELATIONSHIPS AFTER TRAUMA

FRIENDS AND FAMILY

Before the accident, people had always supported me. If I was really sick, friends brought me food. When others needed support, I was there for them. I went to the hospital to visit people, sent cards to people, or went late at night to pick people up wherever they were. I was there if my friends needed me, 24/7. I knew life was hard for people.

After the accident, my parents picked me up from the hospital. However, they didn't rush to get there. This contradicted a few other times I had been put in the hospital in my adult years. I was actually really angry at them. I took a picture of my face and sent it to my mom thinking it would get through to her that I had been hit by an 18-wheeler and was in the hospital. Yet, she and my dad didn't drop everything and come running.

This scarred me. I didn't care that it was a three- or four-hour drive at night. If I had spine surgery in the morning like I had been prepped, I would not have seen them. I wanted to reach through the phone and shake them. I don't know if they were dissociating or suffering a psychological break. Still, their behavior was upsetting and I never forgot it.

I contacted my friends when I got home. At least three of my very best friends never replied when I shared the news that I had been hit by a semi-trailer truck. I tried contacting my friend who lived out of state. However, I received no reply. I considered that she might have gotten

PAIN WITH POISE

a new phone, as that was the quickest way friends could lose contact. I attempted LinkedIn contact. However, I received no word back from her.

I contacted my Columbus friends. They also disappeared. I hung onto hope that eventually they would reappear, but they never did. I was really disappointed in them. They showed me their true colors. I will never understand them. They were always what I considered very good friends. The heartbreak and confusion began. I had left my car feeling victorious and loved, and that I had a life to return to living. However, the life I thought I got to return home to no longer existed.

I tried to be tough, but I needed support. I became really angry at people. They say that just because a person does something for others does not mean it will be repaid. I went through a period of time when I thought about what I had done for others, and I got really hateful about doing those good things for them. Where were they now? I really needed them. I became bitter. I told myself to stop doing good things for people. There was no point in being kind. I felt like I was a really low priority; like I was tiny. I began to fight boundaries and establish new ones.

I had to prepare myself to do things mentally with no repayment. This came with a whole new mentality. Previously, it made me happy to serve others. It was almost a release of endorphins. Mentally, even though I never expected to be repaid, I subconsciously expected it. Now, my subconscious no longer expects repayment. That was a new form of serving. Even saying I would be repaid in heaven wasn't good enough. I was weary just like Jesus on the cross. Jesus was serving others while he suffered. Christians say we are supposed to serve with a happy heart. I don't know if Jesus really had a happy heart that day.

In 2021, a non-medical provider suggested I get a dog trained to help people with post-traumatic stress disorder (PTSD). But it still hurt to bend to do anything. I wasn't going to be able to clean up after a dog due to my injuries. I had not—and still have not—received a diagnosis of PTSD.

LIFE AND RELATIONSHIPS AFTER TRAUMA

It was even suggested that I go to the PTSD trainings with the dog. I didn't want a dog at work. I didn't want to leave a dog at home. The dog would be like having a kid, and I didn't want a kid. Plus, I had considered getting a dog on my own previously and ruled it out for all kinds of reasons. I didn't want to increase my house cleaning either for taking care of a pet.

In addition, those who suggested adding a dog into my life clearly had never seen my calendar. I had no free time. It was like parents when they got their own life after their kids moved out. I had so many medical appointments, at-home therapy, and paying my bills with existing jobs while simultaneously trying to find new jobs. I was seriously angry. Nobody could get it through their heads that the correct answer was LESS. Less work. Less stress. Less responsibility. Less. Less. Less. Less was key to less pain. Less was key to less stress. Less was key to healing.

Then, I encountered people who dismissed my need for "less" because they felt overwhelmed themselves. However, there was a difference when somebody had a sudden disability and their life was centered around healing and coping versus just trying to survive daily life struggles. I used to be that person trying to survive daily life struggles. I really got fed up with being dismissed by people who compared me to them, because they thought they had it really bad.

I became cynical. I became hateful. I became scared of people. Instead of people seeing the good and taking pride in what I was doing right, I was being hammered by people. I had daily battles because of my new health challenges, but few people could see them. Instead, when I didn't do what people thought I should, I was critiqued. I couldn't see why they could not appreciate my daily victories. I was not an alcoholic. I was not at the casino gambling. I was not abusing illicit drugs. I was not driving drunk. I was not suicidal. I was not buying guns and waving them around. To highlight how rough trauma and pain is, some days these were enticing. I would have loved to drink everything away. However, I just held on to the truth that if I moved over the line, it was OVER THE LINE. I held on and slapped myself. I cursed.

A person complaining about trauma is not weak. A person succumbing to trauma is not weak. A person succumbing to pain is not weak. A human can only handle so much. Even Jesus died on the cross. He couldn't withhold the pressure of being tortured. Even Jesus had limitations. I knew one thing: I was not Jesus. I wasn't supposed to be held to Jesus's standards.

One night I was guzzling a bottle of wine like it was water until I realized that it was wine. After that, I decided not to keep wine around. I became very cautious. That did not mean alcohol itself was the drug. I was just thirsty, and I would have guzzled water. As my pain and trauma decreased, I felt fine keeping alcohol in my house again.

Over time, I began to notice that society thought they had a good handle on approaching pain and trauma. However, awareness was not equal to expertise or correctness. They were aware of the need for pain management. They were aware of the existence of trauma. They were aware of PTSD. People also thought all traumatic events automatically caused emotional trauma and psychological trauma. And still others thought emotional trauma and psychological trauma were PTSD. So people compared stories and offered advice. I heard comments like "everyone has PTSD." I was aghast at such a comment. Not everybody has PTSD.

For this reason, I chose to not use the word PTSD. My doctors never diagnosed me with it. I never felt like my life was controlled by trauma. I knew the politics of PTSD. I knew the stigmas. What I endured I observed with curiosity. I called it trauma. My goal was to see how we healed the trauma without the need for traditional mental health treatments. Being hyper-focused on the negative was the opposite of healing. It condemned a person. I had to let go and stop judging myself.

LIFE AND RELATIONSHIPS AFTER TRAUMA

THE CHASM

I maintained contact with my best friend until 2021 when I finally ended the friendship. We had been friends from college. I called her my adopted family. I was in her wedding. She was in my wedding. We traveled together. I even traveled with her family. She introduced me to my favorite beach. She came to my races. Her favorite movies became my favorite movies. Her spontaneous quotes became my spontaneous quotes. I decided to go to graduate school to pursue a doctorate degree in chemistry. She decided to do the same thing at the very same school. We eventually lived in the same apartment complex together through graduate school and we walked to each other's apartments.

When she moved out of state to pursue professional opportunities, we never saw each other again. Soon after, I was hit by the semi-truck and I guess she couldn't come visit. This confused me. I had faced my death and was spared only by God. Yet, she didn't want to see me. I was in bad shape, severe pain, and struggling. I needed my best friend more than she would ever know. I thought long and hard about what she had done. She had still texted me when others had abandoned me. When others made me wonder if I had been a bad person my whole life, and karma was biting me, she still talked to me. Yet, she wasn't visiting me. She wasn't taking the initiative.

I began the descent into wondering if I had deserved to be hit by a tractor-trailer. I couldn't figure out why my former best friend was making me feel so badly. I imagined her out having fun, living her life, while I suffered. We had gone on so many vacations together through our 20s and 30s. I wondered if she had used me and whether she ever liked me. I wondered if she had just needed me for money to go on trips until she finished her degree. Finally, I realized the saddest truth ever. For my health, I had to get rid of her. I was slapping myself. I was not being healthy. I finally said, "You are not my friend anymore." Sometimes crises change people. The chasm was too deep to overcome. We no longer understood each other.

PAIN WITH POISE

I still had great friends, though. I maintained contact with my out-of-state friend Randy, who flew me to visit him a couple of times. I also reconnected with a friend named Gina, from a church we both attended in our early 20s. Since her profession was a counselor, I felt no pressure. She knew I had trauma and she just asked about it. I also felt no guilt. We went to the park and I hung out with her kids. I felt like a normal person around Gina. To my friends, I was still Ashley. We spent birthdays together. Between Randy, Carey, and Gina, I had text buddies. I also made new friends. I still had my long-term friend Jennifer.

As for my family, we didn't always talk through the years. Because I went through so many changes and faced an identity crisis, there were times I took a break from them. I needed time to focus on myself. I needed time to figure out who I was since everything else in life was pulling me everywhere. I needed time to make decisions without their input or guidance. Sometimes I took 3-6 month breaks from them. I would block them on my phone and block their emails. I missed them. But, I had to sort through things. I had to learn more about me. I heard my voice more. Then, it was time to go back to them.

#@!*!*#@*$!

Cursing was a perfect example of being judged. I even judged myself. I never cursed as a child, and rarely cursed until after the accident. When a curse word slipped out, my guilty conscience took over, which was of course due to my societal and religious upbringing. The curse words were a sign of a bigger issue. I could no longer absorb the negative due to the extreme burdens my body was undergoing. I had so much negative inside me from physical and emotional trauma, pain, and stress, that attempting to absorb more stress or pain resulted in an explosion of physical issues.

I compare my releasing a torrent of curse words to that of cursing when breaking a bone. It was really uncontrollable, and quite frankly, using other words that belonged in a world of normal did not belong. Something about this trauma was different. First, I had endured a terrifying nightmare of seconds of pure terror where my body had fought for survival. I also had a brain injury and the added complication of severe pain. This was a tough combination.

I compared the use of curse words to a pressure valve. Curse words for a person with trauma and a brain injury are like mental vomit. Another perspective is that cursing is a brain attack. People suffer heart attacks and people are concerned. Yet, if a person suffers a brain attack, people are not concerned. They are scared. They may roll their eyes. They may call the person juvenile. Pressuring a person to not curse, making a person feel guilty for cursing, or ignoring a person who curses is not accepting of their physical pain.

When a person criticizes the use of a curse word, the person may be criticizing the person for a pain or energy malfunction. For example, if the curse word is due to pain, the person is attacking the pain, such as the nerve pain or concussion. They diminish the pain. When a person curses, that may be the moment they should be listened to the most. By following this theory, occurrence of chronic pain may be reduced. People will be less stressed since they won't need to filter, and doctors and friends will be able to more adequately determine pain levels. There were a few times I cursed when I had adjustments by my chiropractors at Active Edge due to pain.

God knows a curse word includes the torments of trauma. I once met a missionary who said they chose to integrate with inner-city kids by cursing along with them. What an innovative process! Now, the idea was the inner-city kids would never listen to them unless they cursed. As the goal was to get access to them to preach the gospel, they chose to curse assimilate. Christians have this idea that missionaries can pray and then approach a person and everything will happen perfectly. We know this is not true.

Society has been largely unfamiliar with how brain injury scars would materialize. This is why I recommend viewing the person as a warrior. Another perception is to view a person's trauma as a nightmare. A person

PAIN WITH POISE

who has a nightmare screams and curses. That is acceptable. They are forgiven. Forgive people who endure pain and trauma, too.

Sometimes, the real pain and agony of a situation requires a curse word. All other words fail. If I try and use a phrase instead of a curse word, it can inadequately convey the situation or even be a lie. When I can explain it to another person in a grammatically correct form, it's because I am not in a trauma or pain situation. I'm not in hell. When in extreme pain or trauma, it's hell, so I curse. I'm not a Buddhist. I'm not a Scientologist. I'm also not Jesus Christ. This means, I am not perfect. So, I curse.

Cursing also releases energy. It's toxic energy. Explaining it in long form does not release toxic energy. Long explanations also do not release the pain the same way. There is a reason people do not like to be around cursing. It's because it tells the raw, true story. Sometimes people cannot handle the truth. They need it to be filtered.

I had an unfiltered relationship with God. God heard a lot of my "fuck yous." God didn't chastise me. God knew the pain was causing my brain to suffer. God knew the malfunctioning neuron networks were more than I could overcome. God knew trying to overcome it could damage me further and increase my pain.

When I tried to integrate with society, though, I would get chastised. Society didn't know what God knew. What they knew was I was not living up to "cultural" standards of manners, values, and morals. With each chastisement, it was like a rod to my head. I felt the explosion of pain. When I struggled, people ganged up on me.

I worked at companies that employed people who had never been hit by an 18-wheeler. They cursed worse than I ever had. This was why it simply infuriated me to be chastised. I never normally used foul language. To be doing it meant I was sick. This was why I highlighted it to my neurologist after the accident. This was why she said it was okay when I was in pain that I had been mean to people. Use of profanity can be a sign of pain and severe, uncontrollable pain. God knew I was in a conundrum.

LIFE AND RELATIONSHIPS AFTER TRAUMA

When critiqued for my weak moments during my times of pain, I felt like the biggest failure. It was not a constructive criticism. It was not a lesson. It was another stab. I took it as a sign that people didn't actually care about my health. My pain didn't matter. We have all dealt with death. We have all dealt with exhaustion. We have all dealt with loss of jobs. We have all dealt with difficult coworkers. What I went through caused permanent damage. I am still figuring out how to proceed in the future, because I don't trust people the same. Ultimately, intolerance is establishing rules that harm people. Judging people for cursing is just the beginning.

9.
HEALTHCARE HORRORS

After I was hit by a semi-trailer truck, most of my life goals remained the same. However, a few changed, such as retirement. I decided I wanted to retire to the beach instead of retiring to travel. I was going through so much hell that the beach was going to be my final home before I died. I was not going to retire poor and be in debt. My life goals were not going to be replaced with, "I went into bankruptcy."

I struggled with finances after the accident. I faced a lot of fear about how to pay bills and how to survive the future. BWC was supposed to help offset my medical bills, but the MCO wasn't helping this matter.

My first personal injury attorney advised me to not tell people about my accident or my medical concerns. I had to tell my parents not to talk to the family about anything. This was unbelievably odd because my family knew everything about each other. I was also informed the tractor-trailer insurer might hire detectives so I should stop using social media. I was under the belief my attorney would handle medical expenses, as I had heard of credit cards or other medical accounts being used in auto settlements, but this was not the case.

I developed trauma from the IC hearings. From that day forward, everything was fought by the bank that was brought forth by my BWC attorney. I became angry. I once had car issues before a hearing, and I almost didn't make it. My transmission fluid had drained because the transmission plug had popped out. I have learned through the years that transmission plugs can pop out of place due to pressure build-up. Usually,

PAIN WITH POISE

the plug lies beside the opening when this happens. The fluid sloshes out. I said it was like God was trying to protect me from more trauma and pain. Interestingly enough, every IC hearing officer after the first hearing was male. I do wonder if there wasn't rampant sexism occurring.

During this period, I quickly learned doctors would refuse to see a person if they were using BWC. For this reason, my choice in doctors diminished. I was disheartened, angry, and losing hope. I also learned I would need pre-authorizations (PA) for every test ordered by a physician. I would also need a PA to see a specialist. This added time, frustration, and stress. I became even more angry. It took time away from my job for each hearing. It added to my trauma.

My first call for a spine surgeon appointment was refused, because he didn't accept BWC for payment. This spine surgeon was with a reputable group of spine care doctors in the area. I was terrified of the possibility of needing spine surgery and wanted the best doctor.

A year later, I called a specialist when constant rehabilitation was not resolving an issue. She refused to see patients who were being seen specifically for a personal injury claim. She didn't want to be called to court to testify. I was hanging up the phone without appointments a lot. Choices diminished quickly. I was losing hope and getting really angry. I was beginning to wonder why doctors were choosing to become doctors.

One of the reasons I terminated my family physician was because she refused to provide care once I said the accident was going to be a BWC claim. The problem became that the accident was not a BWC claim yet. I had not had a hearing for a BWC doctor to be approved. Her staff could not comprehend that an IC hearing needed to be performed first. I encountered this issue several times. These doctors would insist they were correct, and then I would have no doctor. She implied my expert BWC attorney's counsel was wrong. I couldn't believe she would fight my BWC attorney so much. I was left without a doctor for weeks.

HEALTHCARE HORRORS

After one brutal IC hearing, I was driving to work and saw a semi-trailer truck. I was so angry at the stupidity of the system and the hate that people were using to stop me from healing that I wanted to take the 18-wheeler out. I swerved at it. However, I didn't want to die, and I didn't want the tractor-trailer driver to die, so I stopped. I pulled into work and just sat there.

I was spending years of my life suffering and in severe pain, and the insurers justified destroying me because I was alive. With each attack, someone wanted to physically keep me maimed, mentally scar me, or even put me on the street. I stopped opening mail from BWC. I couldn't read the pain. I just filed it away. I didn't consider it a reflection upon my attorney. After the initial claim, the IC hearing officers were just mean and illogical. What I could not read could not hurt me.

I had an orthopedic nurse from the hospital who refused to wait on the MCO for payment. They were very threatening to me. I had a perfect credit score so I went ahead and paid it, because we hadn't even had a hearing yet to open a claim. I didn't want to deal with it possibly going to a debt collector. I was very paranoid about my credit, so I just paid it. This should have been covered by the BWC neck claim, but they just didn't want to pay.

While my spine surgeon did take BWC, the BWC claim was not approved yet. I paid him entirely out of pocket. The MCO never reimbursed me. I ended up reimbursing myself from my personal injury settlement for both of these bills. In addition, I had the same issue for all of my physical therapy, except for my initial three months of bills.

Not only did I have medical bills to pay, but I still had monthly bills and a mortgage as well. Since I was on BWC, I was repaid fairly quickly by the MCO for my time off work from the bank after the accident. I had to continue living on less money to pay my bills. I was coming from an unfortunate situation where I had not been working for a year for a full-time employer making my normal salary.

PAIN WITH POISE

I had some debt for the first time in my life. Thankfully, I was in a unique situation where refinancing made sense. To reduce this debt, I did something I thought I would never do. I rolled some of the debt into my mortgage when I refinanced from a 15-year to a 30-year. Thankfully, it reduced my monthly mortgage payment.

I also opened a no-interest credit card. I transferred some debt to it and then added new medical debt to it. I did my best to maintain my savings account. My idea was to use a no-interest credit card to pay the bills as long as I could to maintain that savings account. I needed a buffer for a major crisis, such as a roof repair. My savings was there for a reason. I didn't want it to dwindle. I negotiated my electric rates as I didn't need to lock in my gas rates. This saved me a lot of money. By the time of settlement, I had opened several no-interest credit cards.

I also had the added stress of identity theft and fraud. Somebody stole my credit card number and used it two weekends after the accident to buy gas across Indiana. I assumed they stole it at the accident scene, because I left my purse and wallet when I was loaded into the ambulance. Even with cutting expenses, I maintained my identity protection monitoring.

As I was severely restricted in my daily activities, my bills increased because I was eating out more. Planning and cooking were greatly inhibited due to my injuries and disability accommodations. My receipts now included over-the-counter medications like I was filling a medicine cabinet on a regular basis. Those medications were not cheap. I also needed heating pads and ice pads. Friends were recommending essential oils for pain. The list was just beginning. I tried to keep record of these to be reimbursed, but I was unsuccessful.

In the late summer of 2018, I obtained medical insurance for a couple of months to help with medical bills through the bank. This helped until my attorney and I could get everything resolved with the MCO. The MCO moved like molasses in winter. When I chose to resign from the bank, I lost my medical insurance. In 2019, I qualified for medical

HEALTHCARE HORRORS

insurance through my new job at Kohl's and continued fighting with the MCO until I mostly gave up.

In early 2019, I took charge of my own health and started chiropractic on self-pay. I gave up on the MCO and began to see doctors on my own insurance as well. The MCO covered my medications. Of course, the debt increased, but I started getting better. I was no longer waiting on other people or fighting the government. I was choosing the right doctors for me, because I was not limited to BWC doctors. I was finally able to choose a team who followed my philosophy to give me back my health and life.

During COVID, my BWC primary doctor closed. Then, my second BWC primary doctor discharged me for no reason, and I was never able to find another BWC doctor. In fact, when I called the MCO to help me find a new doctor, they started giving me names of doctors in other counties an hour's drive away. I would call and the staff would tell me how to get pre-authorized. Then, they would not send all the paperwork. I'd leave messages at locations and they never returned phone calls.

While the MCO themselves were more than helpful and accommodating in all attempts at connecting me with a new physician, the physicians and medical staff were unable to connect me with a new doctor. I abandoned Ohio BWC. The Ohio BWC system was broken.

Initially, it was the best decision for me to use BWC. BWC did cover the majority of my medical expenses with no issue. However, a person cannot get diagnosed with everything at once. While I was complaining about everything, my doctors were messing up. Things were falling through the cracks. The MCO got ugly. The bank originally promised that everything would be covered, but that was not the case. In order to get better, I had to separate from BWC and BWC providers.

My BWC doctor prescribed my muscle relaxers, but when he discharged me, I had to find a new doctor. I couldn't make it in time, so I tapered myself off the medication. I found a new family physician and

PAIN WITH POISE

gave up on BWC. After discussing everything, she decided it was best to stay off the medications.

I had a feeling I needed other medications to take care of underlying issues, such as the migraine medications I was later prescribed. It's not because they are "bad" for a person, but I didn't want to put more chemicals in my body than necessary. I also wanted to be hopeful that I had healed some. By staying on medications, it felt like I had never healed. Going off medications meant I was healing. Sometimes, when the pain is really bad, I wonder if I should go back on them.

Financially, I did incur a lot of debt over this time, but I was still thankful it was not more. While BWC did pay for physical therapy for the first 3-4 months at physical therapy Location 2, they wouldn't pay for any more physical therapy when I changed locations. I never found out why. I paid out of pocket and I used my insurance. Even with insurance, I learned I had to pay a lot for my physical therapy. Near the close of my BWC claim, my attorney must have finally heard me differently and finally realized I had bills I had paid myself out of pocket.

He said I needed to submit my physical therapy claims, but that was too much stress for me. I was also paying for pain management, such as acupuncture and massage therapy. Thankfully, my BWC doctor wrote a prescription for massage therapy. This made massage therapy a medical necessity.

• • •

In 2018, my personal injury attorney advised me to stay off social media. I had already posted that I had been hit by a tractor-trailer on my professional social media homepage, before I got my attorney. I had friends there and I needed to connect with them about the accident. I was traumatized. I disappeared from my homepage for several months, like he advised. However, he was asking a lot. Did I want to prolong my suffering

HEALTHCARE HORRORS

from a tractor-trailer and cancel my social life for years? No, I did not. I eventually went back to my homepage.

Since I was alone and in so much pain that I couldn't do anything but sit in my house, I decided to stay on my professional homepage. However, I had a lot of males interested in connecting and chatting. I became paranoid. I was afraid every single person who was contacting me on my homepage was a detective. I started chatting with them, though. I wasn't lying about my pain. I hurt a lot. The stress, the feelings of hate from people, and the isolation were all too much. I continued to do the opposite that my attorney wanted. I just wanted to get better. I needed the social interaction; I wanted to be like everyone else! I didn't care about money. It made me really sad and angry that I was being told to sacrifice my humanity and happiness for money.

In the meantime, I was so traumatized that commercials from this law firm made me angry, and I would slap myself. Everything triggered trauma. I left the law firm, and I reported my personal injury attorney to the state's bar association. In all honesty, when I received the letter from them, I didn't open it for years. I just filed it away. I was too raw. I was informed I could sue, but while I was really angry at him, I didn't want to sue him. That was extreme. I stayed with my BWC attorney and searched for a new personal injury attorney.

I had no problem finding a second personal injury attorney. I found that matching one's personality to one's attorney was necessary for a smooth and trauma-easing case. At my final law firm, I was told detectives were very rare and I could go on social media. It was nice because I also didn't feel like I was being watched in real life. I had been looking for detectives in person. I had even been told they might arrive at Kohl's to watch me work. Now, I could regain my life and begin undoing my paranoia. I told my story on my professional homepage, using it like a blog. I wanted to show trauma on professional social media platforms. Trauma was real. Trauma was part of my experience as a human.

PAIN WITH POISE

When a person goes to work, they aren't able to eliminate trauma. Trauma walks in the door with them. Professional social media platforms consist of trauma specialists, physical therapists, and doctors as well as educators who are all interested in learning about trauma from others. They also want to integrate those who suffer trauma into the work environment. I wanted to show companies that humans, real humans with real issues, could work, even with trauma. Companies needed to know what trauma really was.

My new personal injury attorney was fantastic. She empathized appropriately. She provided advice in a hospitable manner. She was soothing. The case wasn't about money when we talked. It was about my health. In fact, she would advise, "Take care of yourself," when I would break down crying. We were a good match.

In addition, I was really starting to feel like anything but myself during this whole ordeal because I couldn't keep a job. I was used to keeping jobs for years. Now, I was walking out the door with an "I quit." I was devastated by my professional portfolio. In five years, I had at least ten jobs. I looked like I was all over the place. In reality, I had a disability that my doctors couldn't figure out, and I was trying to pay my bills. I usually feel people's emotions too much and have to establish a block so I'm not drained by their emotions. With the exposure to predators—both online and off—insurance manipulators, and potential abuse by doctors during a period when my brain was trying to heal, my body and mind began mimicking the environment around me. I was exploding on people over stupid things. I was cursing. I was being mean. I was being irrational.

I began saying things and then felt like I was manipulating people to get what I wanted. I was only doing what others did to hurt me and win. Knowing this was wrong, I began blocking people and isolating myself to prevent hurting others. There were certain things I needed, but my brain was too dysfunctional to ask for them. At the same time, I was trying to stay away from predators. I eventually stayed off my professional homepage.

I also froze my accounts to keep myself from doing illogical things, like sell stock. I wasn't thinking clearly. Selling and buying stocks has an emotional component. This requires skill, and I had a broken brain. I froze my accounts and they hibernated. When I awoke, they had done their thing.

It was brutal going through a personal injury case. The other side has another scenario for everything. I couldn't handle a lawsuit. I thought long and hard about bringing one. However, in the end, it was money at the expense of more trauma. I was slapping myself. I was hating. I had accepted that money was not justice. Money would not undo hate. Money would not undo slaps. Money would not undo scars. I needed to stop thinking and talking about it. I needed attorneys gone. I wanted my life back. A lawsuit would mean more time away from work. It meant more time needing to coordinate my life with attorneys. I said no to a lawsuit. In 2021, we settled.

I still had the BWC settlement. While I thought new claims would come of it, I was wrong. The next few years were spent basically filing the remaining bills to BWC and hoping they got paid. I also was still seeing physicians out of pocket. I updated my BWC attorneys with the latest information and how they were related to the accident. Unfortunately, the personal injury case was closed. However, these could be used to enhance the BWC settlement. In fall of 2022, I signed my BWC settlement. Due to emotional distress, I chose to not file a lawsuit.

However, my financial stress didn't end the day I signed my settlements. I am still juggling real life and trying to find a job that I am able to do that also pays the bills. I am still trying to accomplish my long-term financial goals.

TORTURED NERVES

I fired my first family doctor after having multiple issues with her. She suggested I could do neck stretches before seeing my spine specialist. I had

PAIN WITH POISE

wondered if her advice could be dangerous in case I did have a spine fracture, so I chose to not perform the stretches. I also considered her advice to be disrespectful to the education of other doctors.

This was the same doctor who gave me a horrible time about seeing her because she thought I could only see a BWC doctor. In that case, she thought she knew better than my attorney who specialized in BWC. The doctor refused me care. I'm glad I'm no longer seeing her.

During the first few months of my recovery, I informed my doctors my pain scale was an 8/10 or higher, and they just stared at me. I was suffering real pain, and they were not advising me in any direction that really helped. Pain was taking over. I was losing it. Even after seeing the BWC physical medicine and rehabilitation (PM&R) doctor, I was still in too much pain. All he did was prescribe muscle relaxers.

My physical therapists told me one day they didn't know why anybody thought I was making this up. I was in pain. PAAAAAAAIIIIIIIN. After six months of physical therapy, my doctor wanted to stop and see how I progressed on my own. This was when I flipped out. Part of me thought he didn't realize I was seriously working hard to recover. Part of me thought he was insane. I thought he was stupid. I told him he was fired, and I was getting a chiropractor. I didn't need him. This brings me to my major complaint regarding my initial medical team.

They refused to review me from a whole-body perspective for healing. It was an isolated body part healing, and they would not suggest additional doctors who might be able to help me. I was sorely disheartened. I felt unheard. I felt dismissed. I felt like I didn't matter. In comparison, I had been to other doctors in the past who would advise which doctor I should see for a particular complaint. This prevented stress from research, guessing, and numerous phone calls to find a doctor. After four months of physical therapy under the BWC PM&R doctor, I transferred to MCPC. Dr. Josh Murphy listened to all my complaints and found the source of each. They were not made up or exaggerated complaints. I started to

HEALTHCARE HORRORS

feel less doubtful and more assured and supported. I reported the BWC PM&R doctor to the Ohio State Medical Board. When I looked on the website where he practiced, he had been removed.

In the meantime, I had a BWC family doctor who handled all my follow-ups and referrals. He refused to see me for any of my other issues, so I finally gave up and went to see a new family doctor using my own insurance. When I got to a new family doctor in 2019, this family doctor bent over laughing at my atrophied glutes when she observed my walk.

While it didn't affect my body image, it did make me pause. It made me grieve. I used to have great glutes that were in shape, even when I had a job where I sat a lot. Then, I exercised and focused on conditioning. Now, a part of my body was being laughed at, because it was greatly injured by a semi-truck. I knew my glutes were bad, and looking at them in a mirror put me in a phase of pure horror. However, I was working as hard as I could. This was the nature of the injury. It was neurological. I also felt really weird about the doctor.

This doctor had ordered an MRI. I wanted to get it performed at a cheaper imaging location, but it was too difficult for the office staff to figure out how to process the order. The office assistant became irate. While I stood there, she came charging toward me across the room with her finger pointed at me and told me I was being discharged. They canceled my MRI and discharged me. Even the chiropractor who caressed my knee (See *A Great Betrayal* in chapter 5) didn't discharge me. I was aghast and really scared and traumatized. I couldn't believe that going for a cheaper option got me attacked and discharged.

The office staff said they were going to mail me the discharge letter, but I complained about the attack by the staff member. As I never received the letter, I guess my complaint worked. This doctor's office had their priorities out of whack. I was even stalked on my professional homepage by this doctor's office—totally unprofessional and unethical behavior. I felt bullied and confused, and I believe I was fully enveloped in medical

PAIN WITH POISE

gaslighting by this point. Doctors were fighting me over my pain, not believing the details I reported, and discharging me for no reason.[1]

I compared this to being abused. As I was a very strong and independent woman, I was usually able to brush off most things. While I was proud of my glutes because I was still alive, I was also really angry. What did this doctor do to those people in wheelchairs? Would she laugh at a person with an amputation? I was shaken to my core. What were doctors becoming? I didn't want a doctor like her again, so I decided not to get a new family doctor for my general health needs. I was actually too scared. I put it off for years.

• • •

In the meantime, my BWC family doctor chose to refer me to a BWC neurologist for my neck concerns. I actually had a lot of issues with this neurologist. First, it was upsetting that I needed a new neurologist, because I already had one. This upset my neurologist because she accepted BWC. I heard a lot about this. During the appointment, he talked far too much about my own neurologist. In pain, I was sad and wondering why the doctor was sidetracked during the appointment. It also really made me think differently of my female neurologist he was talking about.

He said he wanted to talk about my worst area since I told him everything hurt. This became overly complicated for me. A person would think this would be easy, but I was so overwhelmed with pain that narrowing down something was next to impossible. Trying to remember and explain different pains was impossible too. I was upset. He also told me it was impossible to have daily migraines. I felt dismissed and unheard by this man. Then, he wouldn't schedule follow-up appointments for my other areas. I was just supposed to call back. This meant I needed to somehow remember this with my stress and concussion issues and not lose it. This meant I would need to get my BWC doctor to do that for me. However, he was very concerned about my brain injury from the tractor-trailer accident and wanted to do follow-up scans.

This was when everything reached a new low. As it was BWC, I had to get BWC approval for the brain injury. My attorney and I were not able to get approval. It didn't matter if the BWC neurologist and my family doctor both agreed that I had a concussion from the semi-truck. I learned the day of the hearing that the trauma unit doctors after the accident incorrectly reported that I did not lose consciousness during the accident. This destroyed my case. There was no justice for my brain, and it was because of one doctor. It had nothing to do with all the other medical doctors who diagnosed me with a concussion. Even Sebastian, the bank's HR specialist, overheard me when I said I had no memory of the accident. Attorneys will destroy a person with incorrect information like that.

I did take backlash for this. I was severely abused and traumatized by some people who found out about this misunderstanding. But I was telling the truth. Sticking to the truth took a lot of brain energy when being abused. I wouldn't succumb to being gaslighted.[2] I couldn't believe people thought doctors were perfect, they never made mistakes, and their notes were flawlessly recorded. I couldn't believe they thought trauma patients were relaying information coherently and perfectly either. People were abusive and cruel to me.

The BWC neurologist also recommended the same nerve pain medications my own neurologist had prescribed. He suggested an increase in the dosage. As I already had an existing prescription for my nerve pain medications, he didn't write a new one. I had been put on the nerve pain medications by my neurologist due to the nerve issues. When I needed it refilled, I went to him. This was during the COVID lockdown so I could not go to the office. While I had seen my other neurologist during this time, I had told her that the BWC neurologist had said he would fill this medication since he had doubled the dosage.

PAIN WITH POISE

I was informed that I would get my prescription sent to the pharmacy upon making my first phone call to the BWC neurologist's office. I gave it a couple of days. I called the pharmacy. They had heard nothing, so I called the office back. This time, I got another story from the office. Since I got a different story, I chose to call back a third time. On call three, I waited a long period of time to connect with a person. On call three, I found out that I was supposed to schedule another doctor's appointment. It had been too long. He wanted to see me again. I could not get in last minute. I was irate. This doctor's office could not follow through with patients. They abandoned them. By the time I could get in to see him again, I would be out of medications.

Stress was high and communication was failing, as I actually could not go and have a chat in person to determine what was happening. I didn't like chatting over the phone. When the staff member returned, she said I needed an appointment. It was rude, irresponsible, and unprofessional of the staff and doctor. He knew he was in charge of my medications and failed to follow through on my appointments. However, no appointment had been made and nobody had told me when to make one, so I had not known to make an appointment. The idea that I would remember to call and schedule an appointment with all of my other appointments, my concussion, and pain was ludicrous.

In addition, I was stunned their attitude was that I was supposed to know the medical jargon and office rules. Apparently, there had been a total breakdown in communication between my doctor and me. Inadvertently, I suffered a serious brain concern while dealing with this neurologist. Here I was during COVID and my doctors were stressing me out. I was having to jump through all these hoops for my basic needs. I was facing medical burnout. I faced fear from having to endure pain because my doctors were living in their own worlds and biases. I was literally afraid I was not going to get my medication. The level of defensiveness from them was staggering.

HEALTHCARE HORRORS

While on the phone, I felt something travel from the left side of my head to the center that felt like a needle and thread being pulled through my brain. This was very alarming. I believe it's an example that should highlight the need for doctors to redevelop management to be aware of stressors. Stressors include tones, words, and conflict resolution instead of escalating situations.

Pre-COVID, this nerve pain medication caused me insurmountable stress every time I went to pick it up from the pharmacy. It was considered a controlled substance in Ohio, so I could only pick it up on the day it was due for refill each month. With pain and not feeling well, this was a lot of effort. In fact, this business was so abusive they had to show how my perspective was wrong and their rules were perfect. They had to attack my self-esteem. The staff was that inept and condescending.

Ultimately, my other neurologist took over my medications. Thankfully, my MRIs came back normal so the needle and thread sensation may have been trauma and not neurological. I had no brain damage. If it was trauma, it was unpleasant news as well. I just know something hit me in the head in the same area during the accident. It left a gash. Nobody ever found any metal in my brain imaging. Could whatever hit me have left a nerve memory of what the impact felt like?

I was so upset that I was supposed to remember all this information and keep it up to date. Then when I failed, I got chastised. A person can only juggle so many balls before they drop one. For me, it causes physical harm and emotional distress. It can trigger trauma. I don't know why the doctors were allowed to do this to me. At some point, medical staff has to say, "This is fine. We dropped the ball." I reported this man to the medical board.

Yet another example of mistreatment by office staff was when I had an appointment get canceled at my local neurologist's office. I had not called to cancel the appointment to see the neurological nurse. In fact, I had taken a vacation day to go to my appointment. However, the staff insisted I had canceled the appointment. I took a screenshot of my phone calls on my phone to prove I did not call. I could have pulled all my phone calls from the wireless carrier. When I asked what number was on the caller ID, their reply was that there was no number.

They blamed the mix-up on my medications and gave me a gas gift card for my wasted drive. I wondered how many canceled appointments there had been, given that they had gas gift cards on hand. I was going to Active Edge multiple times a week, and I did not have one issue with a canceled appointment with them. I never had one of those issues at any other doctor either. It was medical gaslighting at its finest.[3]

I began going to the Cleveland Clinic Main Campus (Cleveland Clinic) to see a neurologist, a specialist, for a second opinion. I didn't need a doctor's referral to do this. I just went. However, this really upset my own neurologist. This then upset me. I could not fathom why a neurologist could not work as a team with a specialist to find the best treatment plan for a person. Instead of focusing on my pain, she was going on tangents, such as taking me off my anti-epileptic drugs (AEDs). I had zero interest in going off my AEDs, and she decided I was a difficult patient. As I refused to see only one doctor, her, she discharged me. I was livid.

This greatly increased my anxiety, because I knew the specialist was only supposed to be short-term. I would need a new local neurologist. I was under more stress. My doctors didn't seem to care about my stress, which meant they didn't care about my well-being. They cared about something else. However, this neurologist also refused to care for my concussion the whole time I saw her, because she insisted *her* neurological nurse[4] was taking care of it. It was a mess.

I was "guilty" of being too decisive and assertive. Medical staff did not get to bully or attack me, because I was both assertive and decisive for my needs. Being a doctor was not a clique. It was not a fraternity, and it was not a sorority. It was a job. They had to accept me. They didn't get to dismiss me the way that they did. They didn't get to confuse me intentionally the way that they did. They didn't get to scare me and eliminate my voice. They weren't allowed to abuse me. We were supposed to be a partnership and a team.

I also had the same normal frustrations as everyone with the added stressors of being sick from an extreme event. I had a multi-year recovery. I was coordinating doctors 24/7, along with the rest of my life. My phone contact list included more doctors than friends. I couldn't even remember my doctors' names.

During my recovery, I considered how house calls from doctors should be reinstated. I thought about this soon after my accident. Doctors used to go to the patient's house. Those doctors really did care. They woke up at all hours to go care for a patient. Thankfully, my pharmacist did make some after-hours phone calls for me. I was scared, because I didn't want the doctors angrier at me. I didn't want the doctors to fire me as a patient. I was literally walking on eggshells with doctors.

Ultimately, good doctors understood that part of their job was to keep the stress from increasing for the patient by making the hard decisions. Did the patient need to stay home from work to juggle all of the medical and legal appointments while healing from their traumas? Was the trauma plus work too much for their brain? Was the patient's brain able to handle the stress and return to work? Were the patient's body and brain able to handle the pain?

When I found a doctor who understood most of this, I started to get better. In a roundabout way, a doctor had to maintain food on their patient's table. If a patient had the ability to grocery shop, then the doctor had to make the necessary life accommodations so the patient could grocery shop. This was why my BWC family doctor helped so much by knowing why work restrictions were so necessary. This was why switching to chiropractic really helped. In addition, Cleveland Clinic focused on eliminating pain more efficiently so I could function better. I also began to take my time and searched really hard for new family practitioners and a local neurologist. I had to evaluate who was appropriate.

PAIN WITH POISE

In 2023, my specialist had questions when needing to complete my Ohio Bureau of Motor Vehicles' Medical Restriction Card paperwork. He wanted me to go to my former neurologist and have her fill it out. Ironically, this was why I wanted to have a local neurologist and a specialist. Specialists can get weird about filling out paperwork. In Ohio, people with epilepsy are required to have a two-part driver's license, which includes a driver's license and a medical restriction card (MRC). My MRC was due to be renewed in 2023. The specialist was the first neurologist to give me one issue with filling out the paperwork, which had been filled out regularly since 1998.

I became very upset. I was currently allowed to drive. In addition, I was the one who had been hit by a reckless driver who had been driving a tractor-trailer. He had a driver's license. It wasn't like I was going around causing accidents or having seizures. I had no tickets. I reported the specialist, and the Ohio State Medical Board got involved. I had to get an extension on my form so I could continue driving legally. I finally got it filled out and submitted. I fired the specialist from my care and my family practitioner agreed that it was in my best interest. The specialist finally filled out the form after advocates became involved and the form was submitted so I could continue driving for 4 years.

When I began seeing my new local neurologist, I was validated. She would've teamed with Cleveland Clinic. I had been right. My former local neurologist had been egotistical and damaging when she dismissed me for wanting two neurologists.

One highly emotionally upsetting and trauma-inducing trend I experienced was the discharges from doctors. As a result, I developed anxiety and trauma related to doctors and their offices. I went to great lengths to find new doctors. I did extensive research. Due to the treatment I received unnecessarily by their staff, I have now become scared of being unable to find medical care. I also became afraid of doing or saying something that would have inadvertently angered staff. When I talked to others who were chronically ill, I knew I was not the only one with similar concerns.

I found myself comparing the medical community to retail. As a professional myself, I really was stunned by the behaviors I was encountering among those in the medical community. Doctors who excelled in their profession had passion for the details, empathy, and compassion. Businesses endured challenging customers all the time, yet they were always welcome. No matter how many times the customer walked through the door they would always be welcome. When it came to people with disabilities, doctors had to excel at their jobs.

If a company sent a letter saying, "You are annoying us. We are banning you. We don't want your money anymore," they would be foolish. That would seem egotistical. That would seem arrogant. That would be bad for investors. This is why I really find the medical community absurd. They want to be a business, but they don't really want to be a business.

The medical community during my recovery showed me it was eager to exclude people. If a patient didn't live up to certain criteria, the patient would be tossed aside. A patient's emotions were manipulated. The medical community was supposed to build emotional health. They were supposed to support their patients. While I had always highly respected doctors, this recovery soured my opinion of them. They caused me a lot of trauma. Thankfully, I now know that it's not just me.

I liked myself. I liked my body. I didn't want my body to be in danger. I wanted my body to be in a restful, meditative state at all times, including at the doctor's office. This meant I wanted to know I was emotionally safe at a doctor's office. Thankfully, I found this at my chiropractors' offices. I was able to recover my mind, body, and soul there. I found it at my gynecologist's office. I am still hoping my new local doctors will satisfy this need. I had a right to be my own patient advocate.

10.
PROFESSIONALLY LIMITED

A person spends 23.8% of their week at work if they work 40 hours a week. Depending on their job, this may be highly repetitive work. It may be highly sedentary, but require consistent typing. It may be a physically demanding job. It is a doctor's responsibility to verify work accommodations will get a patient through the work day safely. A doctor also needs to work with the patient to find a work-life balance for the patient. The patient must have the energy and stamina to be able to accommodate the commute to physical therapy, participate in physical therapy sessions, and then do the assigned physical therapy exercises at home. Keep in mind, all of this is in addition to attempting to maintain other medical appointments, legal appointments, professional appointments, and the demands of the patient's personal life.

My family doctor thought I could easily return to work after one week off work. I protested loudly. I didn't feel physically or emotionally ready to return to work. In addition, I wanted to see the spine surgeon before re-evaluating my health for returning to work. I wanted to make sure my spine was okay. As my family physician had diagnosed me with a concussion and knew I would have an appointment with a spine surgeon, I was livid that she didn't even schedule a follow-up appointment. She didn't alter my work accommodations, either. She advised: "don't move your back" and "don't lift more than 10 pounds." While she did say it may be too much for me physically with lifting and with movement, she didn't consider the mental or emotional toll of dealing with the new injuries or the trauma.

PAIN WITH POISE

Before the accident, I was able to work a nine-hour shift at Kohl's squatting, lifting, hauling, and pushing carts loaded down with merchandise without huffing. Now, I could no longer walk without huffing because of a 18-wheeler. Lifting a pencil was a difficult, painful task. My work accommodations were not detail-oriented enough for the severity of my injuries.

I returned to work full-time at the bank after only a week off work. My manager told me she would not be back to work yet if she were in my shoes. She said, "I'd still be screaming." I said, "Believe me, I tried not to be back to work yet." I was seriously suffering being at work. I struggled through new hire training. While it looked like I did fine, I clearly had a concussion. I struggled remembering new material. All I wanted to do was talk about my accident to customers and employees. All I wanted to do was show accident pictures to people. I was traumatized.

Unfortunately, my full-time job at the bank was unable to accommodate my rehabilitation. By October, I walked out and terminated my relationship with my employer. My final day I was so scared I was shaking from fear because my manager and human resource manager were aghast at my medical requests for rehabilitation. These appointments didn't even include my doctor's appointments. I didn't like their attitudes. I was seriously injured and they didn't care. I didn't matter to them. I didn't have FMLA yet with the company, so I resigned.

When the accident happened, I had three jobs to balance. I worked part-time at Kohl's and Indiana University East, and full time at the bank. At the time, I would have been able to have a work-life balance with all three jobs. I believed in the integrity of hard work. I liked to work. Following my resignation from the bank, my doctor restricted my work hours. This restriction continued until 2020. I didn't want to admit that I needed to reduce my work hours, because I was used to believing hard work resolved issues. However, my body was broken down. It needed rest.

PROFESSIONALLY LIMITED

The only reason the restriction of hours ceased was because my BWC doctor closed permanently in 2020. My new BWC doctor chose not to restrict my work hours. I had mixed feelings about this. Like I said, I liked hard work. Being restricted was hard. I felt like a sick person because I actually had restricted hours. In addition, I did believe it was necessary for me to choose a job carefully that did not require long hours. Therefore, when I looked for new jobs, I did analyze work responsibilities, work hours, and read reviews to get a good estimate of hours expected to work. I am not suggesting a good work-life balance requires work hours be restricted to 8 hours a day. With recovery or even a disability, work-life balance may require a work hour restriction of 40 hours/week or less, 8 hours/day or less, or even how many days can be worked a week.

In hindsight, I found it concerning my doctors thought I could work the same long hours. I could only imagine how many people were not getting adequate work accommodations. A doctor must step in and help the disabled. Working a certain number of hours at my disability level proved to have a negative effect. I firmly believed the medical field failed to understand this except for my one BWC doctor who was really close to the mark. He understood the importance of rest by not only limiting daily work hours but also providing extra breaks at Kohl's as well. This was great because I could not work longer than an 8-hour shift. I do believe limiting my work hours was a medical necessity and should be considered by all doctors when completing medical accommodation paperwork.

While I returned to the shoe department at Kohl's working part-time, my work accommodations didn't cover the extent of my injuries. This proved to be a problem. I pushed apart two shelves one day and screamed bloody-murder. I had no warning I was even going to release a scream. The move generated scream-worthy pain. I had no core or shoulder muscles to brace, but I didn't know that yet. I was moved to the registers where I worked until the fall of 2020. It took roughly six to nine months post-accident before I received accurate work accommodations from my doctors that mostly helped. This was because my injuries were complex. Doctors have a difficult time understanding the dynamics of the human body in movement at work. In addition, my job was very physically demanding.

When I did get more detailed work accommodations, I was in shock at the detail. Work accommodations were broken down to percentages of how many times I could do each motion. Quite frankly, this was guesswork. Who could calculate a percentage of their movements in a day? Work accommodations were a nightmare. Some companies were very lenient on following work accommodations while others were very strict. Through the years, I resigned from very strict companies. It was impossible to maintain work accommodations at places like that.

Navigating work accommodations was proving to be overly stressful. I couldn't believe people really thought we had reached enough of an understanding of my injuries to put it on a piece of paper. Thankfully, my managers at Kohl's told me stories of people being allowed to sit and dust while being on BWC. I knew Kohl's would support me. I was still living in fear, though. I was terrified of bankruptcy and losing everything from the impending medical debt. I was terrified of losing my jobs. It was not guaranteed I would see any money from any insurer if Kohl's decided I needed short-term disability. Attempting to get disability from the government was a horrific challenge. I needed money up front and not at settlement.

Sadly, settlements are not what they used to be. I was advised by my legal counsel that settlements were typically 80% of final bills in Ohio. Some people believe it's really easy to get disabled people what they need in this country. For example, they believe having a disability guarantees disability assistance. In reality, the disabled person meets biases, resistance, and often financial trouble. I had to involve a store manager once because one of my managers didn't understand why I didn't have my settlement within two weeks of the accident. This was a huge frustration.

PROFESSIONALLY LIMITED

People had so many misconceptions, and to educate them would only result in an argument. I had a job with a paycheck, and that relieved some anxiety. However, I began entering a new world in which there was no such thing as rest, escaping pain, or finding a way to embrace disruptions.

My work accommodations said I had to sit. One would think I could sit at a computer for a whole shift, because it was easy for them. Most people would think sitting was a rest break from standing. Most people enjoyed sitting. Most people thought I was really lucky and blessed as I got to sit to work instead of stand. But sitting was not restful for me. It just took a little less energy than standing. It hurt to sit. Sometimes I would stand in pain just to get out of the sitting pain. My spasms would sometimes increase while sitting. However, I had the double-edged sword where complications arose standing. That was the special misery of my life. Everything caused pain.

Basically, I went to work and lived in misery. I would go home and be in misery. Navigating the medical world to have acceptable work accommodations, continually renewing and filing them in order to keep working, and trying to be self-aware enough to know what was causing what issues to improve the work accommodations were developing into monumental stressors. I needed work accommodations that were lenient, had extended expiration dates, or managers who were highly flexible and could use common sense, logic, and flexibility to make their own work environment safe for their employees.

I quickly learned:

- Talking on the phone was horribly painful for the neck and face muscles. I dreaded this task at the bank. Even wearing earbuds for our walkies at Kohl's was difficult to sustain. I ceased wearing my earbud for a long period of time. I still avoid jobs with one.
- Typing involved the neck muscles and was an aggravation as well as very tiring. I was doing putty exercises in physical

therapy, and those were my exercises. This exercise simulated typing, and these very exercises did hurt my neck. I couldn't even look down to pick up Kohl's cash because of the constant up and down motion of the neck.

- My work accommodations could not be written to even accommodate my injuries for working at a register. There is a lot of moving at a register.

This was when I began to become aware of how many pieces there were to the human body. The human body was very intricate. People, including me, underestimate what makes a body function and what is involved when a body moves. People also underestimate how quickly an injured body can fail and fatigue. I could barely function and had to accommodate just about everything. Thankfully, the team at Kohl's stepped in and gladly did a lot of work for me. I didn't even have to ask. They exhibited leadership and inclusion for their disabled coworker.

In addition, my Kohl's coworkers made the atmosphere a fun environment for me to continue to work in my miserable state. This definitely helped me want to come to work when it was difficult to put clothes on or get out of my pajamas. I said, "I've never wanted to wear pajamas all day. I've always dressed, eager to work out and do chores. But, when hit by a tractor-trailer, I finally just wanted to wear pajamas all day." This highlighted just how injured I was, and how difficult and painful it was to put clothes on. It also highlighted how much pain I was in when wearing clothes. It was during this period of time, I listened to a customer. She said she still wore maternity pants, so I decided maternity pants may be a good idea for me. I bought maternity pants. They really did help with the pain.

I also couldn't handle inconsistent schedules at work. My store manager at Kohl's recognized this one day and mentioned it to me. He decided to put me on regular hours. This was a wonderful idea and work accommodation. A consistently rotating schedule was very hard for me to maintain, so moving me to a consistent schedule helped me plan and eased the strain on my brain. It helped the stress. My doctors didn't consider it something that was difficult for my disability, but my store manager had the insight to see a weakness due to my disability.

Instead of just transitioning me to a new schedule, he was upfront and had a direct conversation with me about it so I knew what was happening. I really appreciated his leadership. This was an example of how work accommodations may never be comprehensive enough, and how people with disabilities may fall through the gaps. The smallest detail matters to disabled people. Great managers will be flexible, remain inclusive, adapt, and innovate to accommodate the disabled employee where the work accommodation may leave gaps.

My team at Kohl's was always eager to find a disability-friendly accommodation for me. I had not encountered a team that could handle disability accommodations so exceptionally well. They were highly innovative and empathetic. They recognized handling disabilities of their employees would extend to better caring for their customers. They truly cared. In fact, I was so used to things not working out at other companies and hearing horror stories of most other people's experiences that I lived on pins and needles. I was constantly anxious. Instead, Kohl's opened my eyes in so many ways that showed even I wasn't innovative enough when it came to disabled people.

I learned a novel perspective for successful teamwork. All team members, not just the disabled, were imperfect. For this reason, I learned the value of the team adapting to the disabled. Successful teams want the experience, knowledge, and energy that individuals—even a disabled individual—provide. Innovation merges disabled people seamlessly and positively with the rest of the team, and can be used to improve the company. This was one of the many reasons why I stayed with Kohl's.

Besides having a consistent work schedule, I also required a job with flexible hours so I could schedule appointments for physical therapy, massage therapy, chiropractic treatments, and my doctor appointments. I had multiple appointments a week for hours a week. I could no longer work a set schedule. I also couldn't work at a company that might deny time off or give me any hassle over asking for time off work. I had already resigned from one job that gave me issues over this. At Kohl's, I also didn't have to worry about a person not being able to cover a shift, as somebody was always available to cover my shift. Kohl's was really working out well for me. They also offered excellent health insurance options.

By 2020, I had successfully worked a variety of contract positions. In 2019, my contract ended as a part-time adjunct professor at IUE due to restructuring of the department. My position was absorbed by the new full-time professor. While this position had been mostly online, I wish I could say it was an easy job. With the concussion, pain and trauma, something I had done countless times was even more challenging than when I tutored as a high schooler. This was yet another sign to me that I had a really bad head injury.

However, the position entailed a very different work environment than Kohl's. This allowed me to tailor my work to my needs in a much more individual way. This is also why I chose to work contract positions, such as being a chemistry tutor or secret shopper, through the next few years. These involved much less effort, and I could tailor them to my disability.

Several times, I considered returning to school to get another degree. I began entertaining this idea years prior to leaving CAS, and again right before the accident. I had considered a Master's in Business Administration, among a few other options. Because my accident was consuming my life, I wondered if I should go into medicine. But I can't cut a frog open, much less a human. Plus, I have an allergy to the COVID vaccine so I can't be fully vaccinated. I considered becoming a psychologist, but I really didn't want to hear the worst of some human minds. I considered becoming a pharmacist, but that bored me.

PROFESSIONALLY LIMITED

I decided to get my Bachelor's in Information Technology. I did enroll, but I have not yet pursued the degree. I still weigh my options and still have schools and programs selected. I have even considered going into patent law. If healthy, I would eagerly pursue a new career path with no hesitation. Unfortunately, I have learned that willing myself is not enough anymore. I have a limitation. The doctors were right about one thing: I am young. I have time to wait.

After 2020, I began meeting resistance. Not all companies liked my work accommodations. I was laid off during the COVID lockdown at Kohl's, so I became an employee at an essential company. When I submitted my accommodations at my essential employer, the plan was to put me on short-term leave immediately. I was happy we found some negotiating power. I survived 9 months before calling it quits, though. The accommodation agreements were really too rough. In addition, management would change their minds on how to apply my work accommodations, which made it very frustrating for me. At first, they wanted me to use an electric scooter. Then, they decided I couldn't use the electric scooter. The customers needed it.

Management decided I could periodically use a chair. However, my coworkers did not respect my accommodations. The chair I was supposed to sit in kept disappearing, and I would have to walk everywhere to find it. Then, when it was left up front, the other managers would be sitting or leaning on it and give me issues about sitting on it. They wouldn't get up. I cried every day. Coworkers thought I was just being a lazy employee.

I filed a complaint with human resources for disability discrimination. By the time I quit, it was still under investigation. I ended up quitting because one of those managers said I yelled at her across the room to give her the information she asked instead of walking over to her. I didn't think I was that loud. I was in a lot of pain at this company. I decided the pain and fighting the work accommodations were no longer worth it.

I was also written up at a pharmacy job because I was not responding to somebody. I never heard the pharmacist talking to me across the room. I told human resources I thought the issue was related to my injury, which we were still trying to figure out. I had begun noticing issues with my hearing since we were wearing masks. When we started wearing masks during COVID, I realized I couldn't understand people. It took me a while to understand what was happening.

I was written up for what I considered a hearing issue still being medically determined. I requested a transfer. The transfer was granted. If a deaf person worked there, the pharmacist would have to walk over and tap her shoulder. It was supposed to be a deaf-friendly facility. In the long-term, I received a few diagnoses related to my hearing and brain processing that were disability-related, such as ear nerve damage, migraines, and hemipelagic spasms.

Another time, I was making conversation and asked about a new shipment to the store, and the manager stood up and pantomimed slapping me, right in front of my face, over and over. Apparently she didn't care for my question. No matter how much I practiced positive self-talk, or reminded myself that this was not about me, that simple action took its toll. It was a toxic environment there. I had a manager who ordered me to only look at her when she was talking. I was to ignore everyone else in the room. I felt like a child, or as if I was being ordered around as if I was in the military.

I've had a lot of managers through the years prior to 2018. Abuse is the only word I can use for what I began experiencing from my new limitations. I was encountering one bully after another because I was hit by a tractor-trailer. I was in shock. People were actually mean. I didn't know if I had always been lucky when it came to managers and coworkers, but I was now facing a whole new world of hate. They lacked the leadership I needed. It was affecting my healing.

In one of the companies where I experienced possible discrimination, I was stressed by a coworker so badly that it triggered the worst episode of trauma I'd had yet. In 2021, my coworker was angry at me for helping a customer instead of closing the pharmacy. She was tired and wanted to go home. She was 20 years my junior and said I knew nothing about leadership. I was taken aback that she thought she could dismiss my experience, including my time as a professor. To say what she wanted to say, she followed me around the small pharmacy on her diatribe, raising her voice at me. I felt extremely stressed by her behaviors.

As I had trauma and a concussion combined with pain, I couldn't find the correct words to ease tensions or to move forward. I couldn't think as clearly. I became fearful of this coworker. I started waking up in the middle of the night yelling and screaming in fear of her. This was the first time my trauma had ever escalated to waking in the middle of the night with talking and yelling.

Human resources said I could transfer, but after my experiences at this company I no longer considered them a safe environment for me. I chose to quit my job. I attempted a transfer, but before it could happen my trauma worsened and my job worsened so I walked out in the middle of the job. I didn't care if it looked bad. They made me sicker. They were that toxic for me. I did improve afterward. It's horrible when people at work abuse, bully, or intimidate a person. It leaves scars.

In one online interview during COVID, I suffered a horrendous spasm or trauma attack. I just knew something happened to the left side of my face, and I struggled desperately to keep it pulled together to complete the sentence that I was saying. I didn't even know what the interviewers were doing because I couldn't see them anymore. However, I kept my sentence together. To my horror, the one guy had moved toward the camera to look at me. I was told, "We will let you know if you got the job or if you BLEW it." Needless to say, I did not get that job.

I learned that if God closed the door on a new job, it meant it was a bad match for some reason in the long-term. That made me wonder: What happens when a person has a stroke or a seizure during an interview? Are people trained to hire imperfect people during interviews? I didn't have the answer.

PAIN WITH POISE

After that interview, I became very nervous. Every "Thanks for applying, but you did not get the position," I would get angrier and start to lose hope. I stared at my master's degree and hated it. I viewed it as a stumbling block. It was the reason I could not get jobs. I was overqualified for all these positions. Few saw potential in a disabled person who could not execute at her highest degree. I could not do "this job" or "that job" due to the physical requirements or long hours.

Sometimes, it was the stress or type of job or another issue. Kohl's recalled me from layoff in late 2020. I was offered an internal transfer at Kohl's in 2021, which allowed me to work without needing work accommodations. I was very happy. For once, I got new experience, and it looked like I was doing something in my professional portfolio. Even though I was disabled, I still cared about my professional appearances and climbing the ladder. I was very career-driven. I just could not do it with the simultaneous need to continue healing.

This new position gave me new experience, and I set out to learn the new responsibilities. Kohl's safety protocol set team lifting at 35 pounds, which I could do in a team lift. In addition, this position would not schedule me for freight, so I wouldn't be put in a position that required I do something that was beyond my current health and wellness standards. I wanted to continue working at Kohl's for the ability to have a physical job. My theory was that by doing my normal shift's responsibilities, I could aid my body's recovery by "exercising" it.

During this time, my work accommodations changed. Over time, my weight restrictions increased to 20 pounds. However, my work accommodations restricted my movements in lifting, bending, squatting, raising arms, and twisting. Each movement had different weight limits and different frequency occurrences. There was nothing I could perform at 100%. Most of the movements were to occur at a rate of 0-20% of the shift.

In 2023, I was physically and mentally exhausted. As I was working customer service, the constant contact with customers left me drained.

PROFESSIONALLY LIMITED

It had become too physical for me. Even though my store manager was nice and offered me a chair, I refused a chair. The chair made doing the responsibilities of the job harder. I had started with trauma episodes in the middle of the night, which involved yelling and talking in my sleep, waking me up.

The mirage of lies I told myself in order to keep myself working in a position that was ego-beating was seeping through. In 2017, I had started Kohl's to only help pay the bills until I found my next big dream job. After the accident, it had become permanent. While it was a necessity and it was a wonderful blessing to work at Kohl's, even blessings self-destruct sometimes. I was a sales associate in retail. I was doing the last thing I ever wanted. The job paid bills, and I still learned skills that kept me valuable in the professional world.

Was I still a scientific information analyst at CAS? No. I didn't work for them anymore. However, my skill set said I was still a scientist and an information analyst even if I handled that knowledge differently. I was learning to evolve my ability to analyze information in a new and different manner. It took years, but I became unhappy. I couldn't come up with positive spins any more.

Many people supported me in my search for a new job. However, this was a double-edged sword. I would not heal, and I would lose a job if I proceeded in certain directions. For some people, I did not have a fancy title, such as lawyer or store manager. I was not a scientific information analyst or a director maximizing my degree. I wasn't a pharmacist making tons of money. I finally had to talk to some of them, because they were pushing me to the brink of disaster. Some were criticizing my job choices within a year of the accident. At that time, I was barely navigating medical appointments with professional duties. Years into my recovery, I still needed medical support. I had to get people to understand.

They knew I had it within me to do any job I wanted as they considered me brilliant and talented, but they were remembering me when I

PAIN WITH POISE

was healthy. They also believed the medical and professional worlds were united in equitable platforms to promote a disability friendly culture. I was saddened people were not able to see how I was applying my brilliance and talent to healing from a semi-trailer truck. I had to keep a boundary. I used to be a lot of things. Now, I was part semi-truck. That was my reality.

I believed my self-identity clashed with how others wanted my future to evolve. For myself, I saw a bright future. I saw one evolving as an activist, lobbyist, and maybe a politician. I saw a future where I evolved into a director, president, or a chief executive officer. I was a scientist, and science was everywhere. My future was professionally successful, but it was also active and pain-free. My future continued to evolve so I could be an innovator who could best serve others in this oppressed world. The tractor-trailer could not take that from me.

I was job searching internally and externally. I just could not find a job that worked with my work accommodations. I developed additional issues as I stayed at Kohl's to find a suitable job replacement. I could no longer listen to the music at Kohl's. Even months after my resignation, I was still traumatized by the store music.

I knew there had to be a job where I could spread my wings, and a job that matched my personality better while letting me still heal. I was getting more and more frustrated finding this new company until I finally got a new job in February 2023. However, I encountered several issues at this new company from my manager, so I chose to leave. For instance, a customer complained about my customer service. I was able to perform my job and answer all her questions. She thought I had been slow. My manager had a talk with me and also accused me of breaking a computer. He said I was not in trouble, but he thought I was too sick to work. I felt belittled. I said, "I didn't break the computer. I was not rude to the customer. You don't get to tell me how I feel. I quit." I walked out the door.

I have high hopes of finding the right career fit for my new self. I worked successfully at Kohl's for six years. This showed I can work in a company with my new disability long-term. Through the years, as I supplemented my income with part-time and contract jobs, I also learned more about my new strengths and weaknesses. I learned I was excellent at sales, but I struggled to handle the mentally taxing requirements of planning and organization. I benefited from jobs with little background noise, so I sought jobs that minimized conversations since they might trigger pain.

After the accident, I learned a lot about what works and does not work when a company is trying to assimilate a disabled person. Disability-friendly companies promote cultural exposure in all manners. In order to promote culture, they must be both flexible and inclusive. A disability is a culture. Successful companies know every employee is essential, including those with disabilities. In addition, companies should also be developed to absorb leaders at all levels. This means if a person develops a later disability, and must walk into a company at a lower skill level, it does not mean their skill set is not appreciated. They are recognized for having an amazing skill set, which is not limited by their disability.

These companies must also expand their awareness of how people with disabilities are bullied. People who have limitations are easier targets of bullies, simply because society considers the limitation a real burden. I decided my health matters more than dealing with fake leaders. So, I keep disengaging and pray I can make ends meet until I find the right match for me and my health. One day, I will be who I want to be. I have hopes I can pave the way so others with limitations will have an easier road to achieve their professional dreams in a disability-inclusive culture. I know what I once had in a work environment without limitations, so I know how people with limitations are suffering.

11.
DATING IN THE TRAUMA WORLD

An acute injury impacts all areas of one's life. One's sexual health matters too. So many single people in their newly weakened states are unprepared for the dating world. So many physicians don't caution their patients who are suffering from trauma, concussions, and severe pain about the new challenges they may face when dating. While I had specialists—beyond family physicians, gynecologists, and mental health specialists—who did inquire on paperwork about my relationships within weeks of my accident, they never did discuss them with me.

As it took a few years for me to adjust to my post-accident body, it meant I still believed I could date as I had pre-accident. This was the furthest thing from the truth. As I learned during my recovery that my physicians even struggled to understand the depths of my injuries, it wasn't that far-fetched that everyone failed to be proactive when it came to my sexual health.

I had lost so many close friends. I was dealing with a new bully—pain. To feel like an independent mid-30s adult amidst all my sufferings, I made dating a hobby instead of a possibility. I prioritized finding "Mr. Right."

Unfortunately, I was suffering from a concussion, trauma, and a personality change post-accident. This combination made me put myself in situations that I would normally not have.

I went from being a conservative woman of having only one sex partner, my ex-husband, to one who had a handful. I had some one-night flings. I was stalked. I endured stealthing—a form of rape. I was sexually abused. I was called a "hoe."

PAIN WITH POISE

Even minor encounters with men were majorly dangerous to me. I endured a tickling episode from a guy on a date when I was still unable to wiggle my back. The man was quite aware of my injuries and my recovery phase. My pain-riddled spine and back were still inflexible. When I asked the man to stop, he continued to tickle me with no care for my body.

My injuries prevented me from fighting. With my back injury, shoulder instability, and core instability, I could not even push a man away in self-defense. When I finally realized I was putting myself in tremendously dangerous situations—and this took a few months to realize—I switched to online dating.

Then, I faced the challenges of online dating. What would have been a challenge for any person who complained of their online dating experience was too much for my damaged neural networks. This was when I decided to stop dating. I decided I would just make male friends in real life. As I made friends, maybe something good would happen. By the end of 2020, I was moving forward with healing and focusing on me.

12.
THE EVOLVING "I"

THE BULLIES' DOMINOES

Bullies come in all shapes and sizes.

The horrendous spiritual abuse I endured from the church members made me stop going to church. I began to carefully screen my friends. I had been swatted, ghosted, and shunned. Thankfully, my neighbors supported me through the unnecessary wellness check, and God blessed me with a wonderful friend from the event, but I also developed trauma from the cops. To this day, if there is a knock on my door I refuse to answer. I hide. I don't just hide, I take off running and I cower. I keep my drapes pulled shut. The exception to this rule is if I am expecting my parents—yet I still have anxiety to their knock.

Because of my experience, I became a strong advocate for changing how wellness checks are performed. I believe they are currently abusive and undermine the individual involved. They can be used by people to control a person, to get a desired result, and create an identity crisis in an individual. A wellness check should only be used sparingly, in cases where a person has stated they have overdosed or are known to be missing for over 24 hours.

I thought my days of being bullied by unnecessary wellness checks were over until my disability from the tractor-trailer accident tested society.

PAIN WITH POISE

BULLETS OF TEARS

When I came home from the hospital, all of my neighbors were great. I could come home and be free, suffer from pain, scream, if necessary, and feel welcome. Then, a neighbor's roommate moved back into the area in 2019. When she returned, she began complaining that I was loud all the time. One day, she complained about my vacuum. Our houses were separated. It was as if she were standing at my windows listening. The person she rented from never heard me. The neighbors on the other sides of me never heard me. I know she told everybody about me. She self-diagnosed my issues as PTSD. I always wondered about this woman claiming to hear everything.

This neighbor continued to complain about all the noises in my house. I couldn't figure out how she was hearing everything I did. I started to feel unwelcome in my own home. As my brain didn't handle stress well, eventually my trauma worsened. I could no longer relax, so my pain increased. I began yelling in my sleep. I also left my house so I would not annoy my neighbors if I was going to be in lots of pain.

In the spring of 2022, my hard drive and jump drives began to disappear, which included this very book. I became more and more stressed out. This was horrific for my healing.

Then in February 2023, somebody pulled a wellness check stunt. I was on my final days of my two-week resignation from Kohl's. This was a special two-week resignation to me as I had developed a trend of walk-out resignations after the accident, with few exceptions. I was so happy when I was able to submit one. I had also been dependent on Kohl's and was completely terrified of leaving, even though I had accepted a new job. After the accident, as I struggled with performing at jobs, I didn't think I could do anything else but bag and sort merchandise or run a register. Kohl's had been a stable job as it provided insurance and benefits. I knew my managers from before the accident and they knew me from before the accident. This meant they knew what it had done to me. Still, I was happy

THE EVOLVING "I"

to have planned a resignation with a new job lined up. When a couple of police officers showed up at Kohl's unannounced with days remaining of my resignation, I was devastated. I could not fathom why they needed to see if I was suicidal. I thought they were there for the thieves, because the second I had clocked out in the back, thieves had run right past me out the back door. What the fuck!

To make it worse, the police officers refused to follow the thieves while my store manager chased the thieves. No other police showed up to follow the thieves! These police who were sent to perform a prank wellness check should have become the police who chased the thieves, but in reality they refused. As a result, my spasms were so severe I couldn't breathe, my chest locked up, and I thought I was going to have a heart attack. My happiness and success from overcoming a sick hurdle was tarnished with an attacker's ugly hate of me who called in a false report of suicidal tendency. I was so enraged and insulted that I followed the police out the front door when they left and recorded them on my phone. They did not deserve my respect for what they did to me. I had been a police officer's wife, and I talked to them the same way I talked to my ex. Once outside, I ran away from them. As I ran away, I screamed at them, "Don't get married." Because no woman deserved to be abused by them.

I sat under trees for hours in the dark. The police caused so much trauma and I was so destroyed by the lies that I sobbed and sobbed. I pondered what had just happened to me. I felt watched. Work was now unsafe. I considered going back to finish my final two weeks, but I knew I would be burdened by the added trauma. Instead, I called work and quit that night.

To make it worse, my home monitors recorded them at my house first. Somebody must have told them I was at Kohl's! That was hate. I only knew of two neighbors who would do that. To top it off, they said they were there for an FBI investigation. I don't even understand what they meant by the FBI. Unfortunately, being the ex-wife of a police officer, I knew to be wary of cop buddies doing favors for each other. It was just another instance of bullying a disabled person.

Later that year, I began to see unusually high amounts of law enforcement as soon as I pulled onto the road from my house. I was working a new job at this time. For weeks, every time I left the house, there were cops on my route directly out of my driveway. This was highly unusual. I reported it to the Ohio Attorney General. His office sent me a letter directing me to report it to the correct agency. Then, the police vanished. At night, I would get pulled over for all sorts of reasons. It didn't matter where I went; they found me. Sometimes I was just lost and turning around.

One night I was pulled over by a sheriff's deputy. He said he had seen me not use my turn signal twice and that I had been speeding. I, however, had just pulled out of my housing development. I think he meant to pull over the car I had begun following. The sheriff's deputy repeatedly asked if I had weapons. I had never been asked if I had weapons before. He was so wired, I thought I was going to be patted down for the first time in my life. I was terrified. He was triggering my trauma. I was afraid of attacking since I could not flee. I had two options: attack or find something to hold onto. I was a human. He was a human. Attacking was not an option. Since I literally thought I might die from a bullet for no reason, I began singing "Jesus Loves Me."[1] He let me go—because I was innocent.

In fall of 2023, I got fed up because I was seeing so many cops I could not relax. I was triggered over and over again and could not bring down my stress level. This meant I was in constant trauma. I was sobbing 24/7. I couldn't live normally. This was not helping my facial spasms. My nerve pain would not go away. I was chattering nonstop, because of my left facial pain—the pain can get so bad that I literally cannot stop speaking out loud.

I considered all the unusual issues and came to a conclusion. What I ended up realizing was that my ex-husband had a new boss. His police chief had retired, yet had been hired as the director of a state investigative

THE EVOLVING "I"

unit. And, I considered the new director as shady as my ex-husband. Then, I realized why I was having so many issues with the police. It was legitimate bullying. I talked to a retired female police officer who even agreed with me.

I still feared break-ins. My former manager had shared with me that his police officer father enjoyed breaking into their home after his parents' divorce. For this reason, break-ins never meant it was a random thief to me. I was taking extra steps to barricade myself in at night. Coincidentally, I heard what seemed to be thudding at my front door on several occasions. I eventually saw someone to report to the police, and this person resembled a couple of people I knew in real life.

I posted on my homeowner's forum about possible break-ins and a missing jump drive. I wasn't going to report it to the cops. I struggled to trust the cops now. It angered some people, which was weird, because most people tried to stay away from the cops. I had submitted so many online tips that never got responses, so I no longer considered it worthwhile. However, I was made to feel like *I* had committed a crime. These people were that angry at me for not contacting the cops.

Then, I found out later that a neighbor called the cops to report the theft on my account and said I had been screaming outside. I had not been screaming outside. I was doubly shocked. This neighbor I did not know called the cops for me. He wanted to bully and threaten me with police officers who had guns. He was not really a neighbor.

I told my coworker about the story the next day. Thankfully, my coworker said exactly what my neighbor was. He was a bully. It was an example of controlling behavior. It was also an example of violence. The screams could have been someone goofing off, playing, or even suffering a nightmare. This man simply disagreed with me about how I handled a personal matter.

From these experiences and from seeing the increases in police murders of innocents in the media, I realized each time a person is around a police officer, they are around deadly and dangerous weapons. They carried tasers.

PAIN WITH POISE

They carried mace. I no longer trusted the police to make sound judgement decisions. My life was precious. They could kill me based on their perception of my semi-truck injuries, and that terrified me. I didn't want to die because a police officer thought trauma was danger. I didn't want to die because nerve pain and spasms looked threatening to a police officer. I didn't want to die because I wanted to get in my car and drive to the park due to nightmares. It was time for a change in law enforcement and any interaction with human beings. I was living in terror of dying because I knew that cops pulled guns on people they should not pull them on.

The unsupportive neighbors chose to "help" by intimidating a person to fall into "order" by calling the police. These neighbors chose to terrorize a disabled person using police officers who had guns and handcuffs instead of socializing or dropping off food. And this was not just with neighbors. I believe this applies to anybody who calls the police to override a competent person. The friends and neighbors chose intimidation with the risk of death by simply putting their friends and neighbors closer to a gun. I love my friends, family, and neighbors. I don't want them closer to a gun. I want them far away from guns.

All of these police encounters led to paranoia. I was glad for the law enforcement presence, especially as crime was increasing in the city. Yet, there was a tug-of-war every time I saw police officers. My gut told me somebody was paying inappropriate attention to me. In fact, I stopped to talk to the sheriff and he verified the higher crime area pulled the police from my area. The police would not be in my neighborhood. I felt justified in my fears of being almost stalked. Seeing and hearing the sirens from the police vehicles was breaking me down and wearing me out. I was determined not to change. I was still in a delicate phase of healing, and I was livid I was being destroyed. I needed to take a break from police so I could breathe and heal my overstimulated nerves, emotions, and brain.

With trauma and PTSD comes prejudice and stereotypes. People would manipulate the "fear" and current events to intimidate and coerce people. For instance, people with trauma and PTSD are supposed to be violent. Apparently, society also thought people with trauma and PTSD were going to commit suicide. Then society thought the answer to suicide was to expose the person to people carrying murderous weapons to force them to conform. Enough! These sadistic cycles must end.

These bullies plant seeds. If society believes a person with trauma has guaranteed traits because of their existing trauma, then they doom the person. The stigmas associated with trauma and PTSD are so damaging.

When I thought about what was happening to me through my recovery, I finally decided it was like people wanted to sabotage me. I decided people were angry that I was healing. This was a great reminder that people have to resolve their own issues. I couldn't force the other people to fix their issues. My problem was healing and recovering from a semi-trailer truck accident. When it seemed like people wanted to sabotage me, I chose to leave. I chose to walk away. I chose to disengage. Then, I got to try and find a place a cop wouldn't show up. As such, I am now back to sitting in my house with my drapes pulled. But, the cops can't look in. My neighbors can't be nosy. It's all mine.

PRO-CHOICE IS RESPECT

After the tractor-trailer accident, I suffered. I lived in agony. It was a unique agony and an indescribable suffering. Pain was a bully. So, I made a decision: If it ever came to extending my life or choosing death, I would choose death. If I lived in a world where assisted suicide was freely an option for any reason, I believe I would heavily consider it. Living with pain and trauma is a curse. Living in a world not open to the disabled is a burden.

I also consider our current methods of suicide awareness a form of religious persecution. Not everybody is as religious as the next person. This country is founded on religious freedom. As much as I am a Christian,

PAIN WITH POISE

I am not here to force my religion on my neighbor. I don't enjoy forcing my politics or choice on other people either. I don't like controlling other people. I am here to respect my neighbors' decisions. This is why I choose to be pro-choice for people's end-of-life wishes.

13.
THE COVID-19 PANDEMIC

When the COVID-19 pandemic struck, I was forced to change my recovery team. My gym, acupuncturist, BWC doctor, physical therapist, and massage therapist were all closed to patients. I remember sitting in shock at the news of losing my support teams. I even took a picture of my physical therapy team on my last day before lockdown.

How could medical professionals close? How long would they be closed? My pain was crippling. I had the foresight to see a disaster where a lockdown would be months and not weeks. I was a scientist, I had amazing history teachers growing up, and my dad raised me to understand how the government works. I knew we were in trouble when the government did the lockdown.

My trauma worsened. I was livid. Medical professionals were closing their doors in this country. The excuse was we had never encountered a pandemic coronavirus before, and we didn't know how to wear masks. Like I said, I'm a scientist. I don't have much anxiety. Just put on a mask. I went out and got a job. I know people died. I had family who died. Yet, my very family almost got a phone call that said I was dead from an 18-wheeler. Sadly, a lot of families do receive that phone call. Death is death. For this reason, I didn't understand why my medical professionals were being ordered closed.

I was still alive. All the fearful people silenced my voice again. All the powerful people silenced my voice again. I was a nobody who was living in horrendous, scream-worthy pain. I became desperate. Was I

PAIN WITH POISE

really supposed to suffer? Basically, yes. During the lockdown, I was told I was supposed to suffer and medically worsen. Even though I had a basic human right to health and wellness and continued recovery, I was told I was not allowed to access that right.

I was not going to sit at home and suffer while people abandoned their medical duty. This was disability discrimination at its finest. With each closing place, they insinuated my pain and suffering did not matter. I didn't take that well.

During the lockdown, the healthy people got to go home and turn it into a game. They enjoyed working from home. They got to stay in their pajamas all day. They got to watch movies all day. Some people lost their jobs, but many received unemployment benefits. Yet to me, the lockdown and the closings meant staying in (increased) pain as my own medical teams closed their doors one by one. I was supposed to lose my support group because of the government. I was supposed to lose all ability to do my physical therapy exercises that required equipment because of the government. People like me simply didn't matter.

I was okay with waiting a week for my therapies or pain treatments to resume. However, I was not willing to wait weeks or months for my brain to be damaged further by chronic pain. I was not going to be abused by pain. Erik Hensel, D.C., at Active Edge even told me that chronic pain results in damage to a person's brain. I believe the lines blurred and society refused to accept that this decision was an act of neglect against a large group of society. And I believe those places that decided to stay open are true medical providers. In addition, there were negative consequences of the lockdown on people needing preventative pain management. These treatments were not always adaptable to the home. For example, chiropractors were not walking to patients' homes. Physical therapists were not delivering weights and other fitness equipment to clients' homes. Therefore, when medical businesses closed, people were losing their resources for pain management.

THE COVID-19 PANDEMIC

When this happened, a person's risk for needing the emergency room may have increased. People may have needed pain medications or they may have gone to the emergency room for falls or injuries while trying to do physical therapy while not monitored. As some research indicates, the injury severity score of trauma accidents during the COVID-19 lockdown increased. While visits to trauma and admissions greatly decreased, and overall injuries decreased, Arastoo et al. (2021) found reports of concussions, hip fractures, and ankle sprains increased. Suicide even increased during the COVID-19 lockdown as 23% of the severe traumas were suicide attempts compared to 2% before the COVID pandemic.[1]

Those who suffer from pain may be more hopeless and sad, especially when they are told they do not matter by the government and medical centers that close. Therefore, shutting the doors on medical facilities to aid people in pain management was an unwise decision. This cause and effect was very concerning to me. As a person suffering from pain, I was shocked that our government and healthcare systems had made these horrifying decisions.

Additionally, people lost their coping mechanisms and support groups. Prior to the lockdown, I would leave my house and go to my local grocery store, which was open 24 hours, to deal with my pain and trauma. There was nothing better than shopping therapy and being around people to stay engaged. It was nice to leave the house at 2 a.m. and go to the store and walk around and be bothered by nobody. I could talk to nobody and just look at the pretty things. I could dream and browse and remember what I needed to do at home. I thought of projects and bought ingredients for meals. It was a healthy habit for me. It was better than sitting at home drinking or hating or watching violent movies or screaming.

At the store, I also had to make myself control the screams. I was still in pain, and I was still in scream-worthy pain, but there was an added layer of healthy stress and training that required I stay poised in public. At home, I would get angry. At the store, I would stay calm. How does a person get angry when she is shopping and isn't failing at exercises or triggering trauma during physical therapy? It's hard.

However, with the closures, my coping mechanisms were destroyed by the COVID-19 lockdown. They were not destroyed by COVID. COVID was a virus. The only thing that blocked me from 24-hour stores was the government. When I had pain and trauma that was so bad it would literally be suffocating at times, I was too scared to sit at home alone. When my body parts were neurologically weak and not functioning correctly, I wanted to be in public. I wanted my support groups and my coping mechanisms to be normal. It was too much for me and my disability. Finally, another reason finding replacements was necessary was because I was not healthy enough to do my exercises for weeks without supervision. I could seriously injure myself.

I began writing to my politicians about lockdowns and ways of managing health and wellness. Thankfully, the state of Ohio allowed an exclusion for health and wellness, which allowed me to leave my house for medical treatments and for physical outdoor exercise. I maximized this exclusion and got out of my house every day to walk and get a change of scenery. Changing scenery was vital for my mental health.

With the announcement of the lockdown, I immediately began searching for replacements for my gym, acupuncturist, and massage therapist. At the time, I didn't know if I needed a replacement for my chiropractor. I was able to find a massage therapist who would travel to my house. She said I fell under the exclusion called "helping a person in need." I found a new acupuncturist who treated only severe cases during COVID-19. She considered me medically necessary. Once I found these two replacements, I started looking for a replacement for physical therapy. I specifically needed access to a Bosu ball, fitness bands, and an elliptical. I recalled one of my chiropractors from a few years prior who had a great gym setup. I sent an email to them. I impatiently and frantically waited.

THE COVID-19 PANDEMIC

When I switched to a chiropractor in 2019, I had not returned to my go-to chiropractor—Active Edge—because I wanted to try a different chiropractic method for my cervical neck adjustments. My neck was so painful that I could not foresee causing it more pain with a quick neck adjustment. I admit I had not been to a chiropractor since 2015 as I had felt healthy. Yet I knew from experience that Active Edge chiropractors cracked the neck. That's all I had ever known they would do, even though I was familiar with other chiropractors using other methods. Through the years, I had also grown a bit concerned about quick neck manipulations after doing some reading and having a neurologist caution against having them performed. I assumed this quick neck manipulation was the only technique Active Edge would use on the neck. These reasons encouraged me to go another direction in 2019 when I decided to add a chiropractor to my medical rehabilitation. Dr. Josh Murphy at MCPC became my chiropractor when I learned they used gentle neck manipulations.

The morning after my email to Active Edge, I received a reply from Jasmine Craner, D.C., C.S.C.S. I was extremely happy. Dr. Craner explained that I was able to receive unlimited chiropractic services and a few other services with their Life Activated Partnership (LAP). The LAP guaranteed the monthly rate for life. The initial agreement required a one-year commitment that could not be cancelled. After the first year, the partner was able to cancel their LAP at any time, but they would have to rejoin at the new LAP rate instead of maintaining the lifetime rate from their first LAP. This also gave me access to the essentials I needed to continue with my physical therapy, except for an elliptical. I agreed.

Upon my initial consult, Dr. Craner determined she needed to see me two times a week. This doubled my chiropractic appointments from my chiropractic treatments at MCPC. As I had joined as a partner, I didn't mind. I was curious as to what the change would be in my recovery between the two chiropractors. I was also curious in how the chiropractors might complement each other.

PAIN WITH POISE

She wanted to crack my neck. I decided to let her try. The pain was too intense. She had to do some muscle manipulations to get my neck to release before it would even move. Then, I would brace. The fascia was so tight and inflamed that I grimaced against the pain. She could only manipulate one side of my cervical spine with her hands.

Then Dr. Craner introduced me to other methods to adjust my cervical spine. One very painless method Active Edge's chiropractors used with me was an activator. An activator is an instrument that produces a quick, low pressure thrust that delivers a controlled force to adjust spinal joints. This method allowed my neck to stay in a neutral position while the chiropractor adjusted my cervical spine. My cervical spine was also adjusted with a drop piece. A drop piece is a part of a chiropractic table that slightly drops allowing the chiropractor to more gently adjust the neck in a very controlled manner. Another method to adjust my neck was used after my eye surgeries. Dr. Craner had me sit in a chair since I could not lie on my back during my eye surgery recoveries. Now, I have my neck cracked every time I have an appointment with no fear.

I cheered the day things improved and Dr. Craner was finally able to adjust both sides of my cervical spine with her hands. It hurt so much I had to rest between manipulations and bite back curses though.

Dr. Craner encountered the same issues when attempting to adjust my back. From the very beginning, she couldn't perform all manipulations on my back. The sensations felt like bruises with each compression of her hands against my body. However, the pain very slowly began to diminish as I continued my frequent appointments.

In the spring of 2020, I decided to try running. I had been using the elliptical for exercising at the gym, but I no longer had access to one. Even Dr. Craner thought I would be fine with running. So, I went running for a short distance. I thought it had been okay. Afterward, I couldn't make it down the stairs. My right knee was destroyed. It was unstable to the point it hurt to walk on a flat surface for weeks. I had to wear a knee brace for months.

THE COVID-19 PANDEMIC

I stopped running and my new medical team went back to re-evaluating my injuries. This cycle was how we progressed over the next few years. I would try an exercise. I would state what I felt, what was not working right, what was too difficult, or what I could not do. My team would review it and do some physical tests, make some adjustments, and then advise me in therapy corrections to attempt to eliminate those issues.

While everything was going great with my chiropractor, my medical doctors were starting to fail me. My chiropractors created a safe and non-stressful environment. It was a happy and positive location. I looked forward to my visits. However, in the summer of 2020, I was trying to have a phone appointment with my BWC doctor and something went wrong. I was sitting there, waiting, and still missed my appointment. I called the office and spoke with the staff. They were not very nice. They were usually very nice on the phone. I was blamed for missing the appointment. I didn't appreciate being wrongfully accused. I needed work accommodations for my job to be updated. I didn't want to lose my job.

Then, one day, the staff said I was discharged and the practice closed the doors permanently. I lost my BWC doctor who did all my paperwork. I lost my doctor who wrote my prescriptions for muscle relaxers. I even lost my doctor who recognized why I needed a prescription for massage therapy. I lost him because of COVID distance.

COVID distance, a term I made up myself, is a barrier where one is forced to communicate using the Internet, telephone, or mail. COVID distance eliminates the easiest form of communication: in person. Facial expressions are lost in mail correspondence and telephone conversations. The tone of a person or their message can become harder to clarify, depending on which form of communication is used. Communication breaks down due to COVID distance.

With the closing of my BWC doctor's practice, I became even more stressed. Thankfully, my attorney recommended a replacement who

PAIN WITH POISE

accepted me. Then, I tried to get a refill from my neurologist that I had seen for BWC.

During this time, I drove by the chiropractor's office that had treated me in 2019. It was to my horror to see a faded business sign and empty office. MCPC was gone. My personal injury attorney had also explained she was having difficulty contacting Dr. Murphy to get my medical files for the settlement. I was terrified because I thought they had permanently closed. Thankfully, I eventually made contact with Dr. Murphy after the lockdown was lifted and learned they had only moved their business to a new location during the COVID lockdown and had indeed stayed open to treat patients. However, there had been a lot of confusion due to the disenfranchised state we had been living through during the lockdown.

I had additional complications during the COVID pandemic. My retina detached in my right eye in summer of 2020. There is nothing quite like needing emergency surgery during the COVID pandemic. It was essentially go blind or have surgery ASAP. Thankfully, I passed the COVID questionnaire and wore a mask during surgery.

In addition, I learned I had experienced what seemed to be an allergic reaction to my vaccine. I had to take an antihistamine to stop the side effects I was enduring. My specialist called it an irritability. My chiropractor put me on a detox. I reported the issue to VAERS. Unfortunately, I can't get any more vaccines. I am one of those people who can't be fully vaccinated. Personally, I am against vaccine mandates because I am a scientist, so I am highly aware of allergies and how chemicals affect a human body. I have met people with the strangest allergies. I also know to always err on the side of caution. This means to put the power in the hands of the people. The people have the right to decide for themselves what goes in their body.

When the COVID lockdown began, everything looked dire. Yet God opened a door that put me on a new journey to reclaim my body and health from a tractor-trailer accident with the use of functional medicine.

THE COVID-19 PANDEMIC

By the time the lockdown had ended, I had a medical team that was working, and it was radically different from my pre-COVID lockdown medical team. I was even inching closer to my accident recovery goals. Yet I was sadder because the America that I loved was gone as my rights had been restricted with lockdowns and curfews, people were still attacking each other over stupid masks, and people literally hated people who had opposing ideas.

14.
ENERGY, RESEARCH, AND INTELLECT

UNRAVELING THE PAIN

As a scientist, pain means something is wrong with the body. During my recovery, I was introduced to a society that judged people who were in pain. One reason I believed this was the case was that society largely believed people complaining of pain wanted narcotics. In fact, I had a discussion with someone who had a similar pain situation and repeatedly went to the emergency room. She was continually treated rudely because they thought she was there for narcotics. This was not the case. Society also refused to recognize pain as real. As such, they were failing to properly diagnose people for what was causing the pain. I had to establish brick walls that were miles high in order to stay true to myself. This only worsened my recovery.

To rehab my body, I encountered a major problem. Somehow, I had to build each body part without the use of other body parts. Conventional techniques used too many body parts in a single movement. Because the body is interconnected, this posed a problem. For example, core muscles are connected to the neck muscles. Fascial lines connect the leg to the hip to the core to the neck. With a destroyed core, I was having to rebuild my core and rebuild the lower and upper segments. I couldn't do upper body exercises that involved my lower body. I couldn't do lower body exercises that involved my upper body. When I attempted to do an exercise that involved both, I was not able to engage my core or glutes.

PAIN WITH POISE

I described my body as "a shredded body" because that was how it felt. To heal it, we needed to treat it with more than just surgeries, bandages, and ointments. In hindsight, I had a very complex injury. Not only was I dealing with a cervical herniation, but I was dealing with other injuries from head to toe involving a concussion, multiple micro tears of muscles, sprains of ligaments, and injured fascia bands. Eventually, I learned how badly the fascia bands were injured.

Fascia bands are connective tissue that wraps everything in the body. It is tightly compacted and wraps around individual muscle in order to connect it to other muscle. It wraps around bones, tissues and organs. Fascia even wraps around blood vessels, nerves, and arteries.[1] The fascia chains do not go up and down the body or around without crossing each other. Instead, the fascia chains crisscross and even attach at opposite ends on opposite sides of the body at times.

Dr. Craner compared fascia bands to rubber bands. Imagine an elastic rubber band (fascia band) secured around two poles (muscle). When injured, tears and inflammation result, causing scar tissue (adhesions) of the fascia. These adhesions create tension within the fascia band.

This tension will then cause distortions in the surrounding organs, tissues, and muscles. One well-known result of damaged fascia are trigger points in muscle. A lesser-known result is nerve damage. If the adhesion is farther away from the core, it will trigger fewer issues within the body than an adhesion closer to the core. This is because of the large amount of fascia bands in the core versus in the extremities.

The goal of treatment was to determine where the knot was in order to eliminate the knot in order to heal the fascia band. These adhesions of the fascia are like dominoes cascading within the body. Unfortunately, when one adhesion forms, there is a dysfunction in the body which may result in pain. The body will adapt to offset this dysfunction by causing another dysfunction, altering in structure.

ENERGY, RESEARCH, AND INTELLECT

Dr. Craner explained the possible injury scenario. The fascia chain's job was to save life. One fascia chain would have connected from my toe to my neck and tightened to keep a bowling ball (my head) attached to my neck. The fascia band stiffened upon impact to be almost cement-like or cable-like to prevent my neck from moving beyond its normal position. In addition, my accident involved a multi-directional hit and not one directly from the back. This multi-directional hit then involved multiple fascia chains, so it was no longer a uni-chain injury. Therefore, each fascia chain involved in the accident would react the same and become damaged. As Dr. Craner explained, "If an (high-impact) accident forces fascia chains to activate that cross mid-line, or the center of the body, it becomes more difficult to treat the injury, because the injury involves multiple chains." Therefore, my accident resulted in a multi-fascia chain injury.

Since modern medicine has a tendency to compartmentalize body parts, traditional therapy sessions were missing the aspect of the multi-lateral complication of fascia chains, connected muscle, tendons, and more. Just like the chiropractor, the therapist knew there was a relationship between the neck and a finger, and recognized the relationship between the neck and the core. While they recognized fascial bands and chains were involved, the therapist still treated them differently than the chiropractor.

Another complication arose when everyone wanted to start me at a level too high for my body to handle. Some people didn't consider I had a back injury. They were beginning me at a level that should've worked if I had a cervical herniation from falling off the couch or slipping down a hill. I would've had a healthy, functioning body everywhere else to support the exercises. However, this time I did not. My entire body was wrecked.

In addition, I was weak. I fatigued quickly unlike before the accident when I exercised daily and ran. I ran several days a week. In fact, I couldn't just sit at the house and do nothing. When I was hit by the tractor-trailer,

PAIN WITH POISE

I received an instant new body. The energy from the semi-trailer truck had shredded it. My team had many challenges unique to this recovery, I surmised, due to it being an extreme impact accident.

While I complained of my pain level for years, I had to fight to get medications to treat my pain. In my strongest, and most educated opinion, I believe my doctors chose to under-treat me for pain and inflammation. At first, all I was advised to take was over-the-counter medications to help with pain.

By late 2018, I was prescribed a prescription for muscle relaxers. However, these were not sufficient. I supplemented these medications with more over-the-counter medications.. Eventually, I was prescribed nerve pain medications. Finally, after much research and patient advocacy, I received substantial prescription support for migraines.

My medication list:

- **Year 1**: Maximum dosage of over-the-counter (OTC) naprosyn; OTC ibuprofen; OTC acetaminophen; prescription muscle relaxers; topical essential oils; topical pain relief ointments
- **Year 2**: Prescription nerve pain medications; increased dosage in muscle relaxers; daily use of OTC acetaminophen; sleeping aids
- **Year 3**: Prescription migraine medications; aspirin; OTC migraine medications; sleeping aids
- **Year 4**: Increased dosage of prescription migraine medications; OTC migraine medications; sleeping aids

I averaged 1200-1600 mg of ibuprofen every day for the first few weeks. I was on acetaminophen every day for years. I finally stopped taking acetaminophen, because my nurse said it was bad for my health. I was to decrease taking it. Therefore, I ended up just suffering. I was prescribed medications for nerve pain. While it helped some, it was not taking care of my only pain. I also began taking supplements with fish oil and ginkgo biloba to help support my brain from the stress and the concussion. I took supplements to support joint health, such as glucosamine chondroitin. I took probiotics to support gut health.

Post-accident, I had irregular bowel movements. Before the accident, I had always had regular bowel movements. Therefore, I was concerned this was a side effect of the trauma from the accident. In addition, I learned the gut also had a connection with the brain. I began taking probiotics. After extensive chiropractic treatments and rebuilding my core with the breathing techniques, my bowel movements returned to normal in 2022.

Eventually, I tapered off the nerve pain medications as my doctors and I decided it was not the best fit for me. I didn't like how I was feeling on them, and overall, I didn't want to be on the medication. It was also a fairly small dosage. I also tapered off the muscle relaxers. I really wanted to test going off the medications to see how the chiropractic was going. My family practitioner thought this would work well.

TRAUMA AND PHYSICAL REHABILITATION

While chiropractic and functional medicine is what ended up working for me, that's not how my recovery story began. I began with traditional physical therapies, which compartmentalized my injury. The more I attempted physical therapy, the more I suffered. In addition, I began physical therapy when I was just learning my new body. Therefore, I incurred a lot of trauma during this period. I incurred trauma because I learned how damaged my body was, and I incurred trauma from the physical therapy. I also learned that my body became more inflamed from the exercises.

I had high hopes when I entered physical therapy. Unfortunately, physical therapy went anything but smoothly. I walked into physical therapy Location 1. The heat therapy was nauseating. My therapist said he would have me sweating in no time. He explained his plan and I seriously

PAIN WITH POISE

doubted he understood my injuries. I switched locations.

At Location 2, I encountered extreme pain. My physical therapists advised me to go to urgent care so urgent care could handle my pain after sessions. That was unacceptable. A physical therapist should not put a patient through treatment that increases pain to the point of seeking pain treatment. I remembered driving home one day after an appointment where my left arm was propped against the door because it was searing in pain, and I was crying. I couldn't use it to drive.

In the process of learning what pain was, I endured a lot of suffering. Then one day, the new physical therapist at Location 2 wanted me to try the rowing machine standing. I told her I wouldn't do it. I knew it was wrong for me. However, she refused to listen to me, and said she knew best, so I obliged. I did a half rotation and I had white hot pain raging through my body and brain. I could've ripped her in two pieces with my bare hands with the animalistic pain that overtook my body. I left and went to my BWC doctor. My blood pressure was still elevated hours later when the doctor took it.

As my physical therapy progressed, I learned to hate the paperwork assessments I was supposed to fill out. For starters, the doctors didn't care about all of my injuries. They were hyper-focused on my neck. Secondly, I learned I couldn't adequately highlight how I felt on the paperwork. I thought about how this could have happened. I considered that I was delusional as I was not accepting reality. I considered it was my concussion making processing more difficult. I considered that I had been overwhelmed by the paperwork. I also considered that I was wrongly assessing my body, because my doctors kept ignoring my complaints. I came to hate the paperwork. It only told part of the story.

I wanted to heal the parts of my body that were hurting. It took a year for me to get a doctor to finally agree I had lower body injuries from the accident. This only validated my feelings that doctors didn't care. It made me feel doctors were only in their jobs for the money. If I didn't continue being my own advocate, my body was doomed. The problem was

ENERGY, RESEARCH, AND INTELLECT

I was running on fumes. My body and brain were damaged and tired. I was not able to be as strong as I normally could to fight for my own body. I was at a horrible disadvantage trying to fight for my health and rights.

I couldn't just listen to the doctors and proceed while knowing something was not right. It was like I was not supposed to have these injuries, or I was supposed to be better already. I felt a lot of pressure from people when my injury didn't heal in a pre-determined amount of time. It came from some of my doctors, physical therapists, attorneys, and insurance companies. In a way, I felt like I was supposed to be completely healed within three months.

As this wasn't the case, I just stared at people as if they were crazy when they offered an objection. As a human, I knew my body. It wasn't healing. As a scientist, I had an analytical brain. It made sense to me that the body needed more time to heal, as I had multiple injuries and I couldn't fix them all at once. I knew physics. I understood engineering. To me, between what I felt and what had transpired, I had a long road.

For anybody, it would be extremely frustrating when others told them how to feel. It erodes a person's confidence and exhausts the person. As such, the very people who were supposed to be working to heal and build me back up were ultimately tearing me down. Insurance companies, doctors, and attorneys were focused on speed. My injuries were not localized to one body part. It was intricate and complicated.

I couldn't let the doctors gloss over my injuries. I couldn't let my physical therapists gloss over my dysfunction. I had to do something ugly. I had to stop and examine every pain, ache, stiffness, and pattern in order to find the answers to heal them. To recall all the pain and injured body parts would bring about trauma and extreme emotions I could no longer tolerate. It would bring about confusion. It was exhausting, debilitating, and depressing. My brain was overloaded. It was trying to recognize the severity of my debilitating injuries. A piece of paper no longer worked. It was beyond circling. It was beyond arrows. It was a whole-body injury.

PAIN WITH POISE

It could not be simply explained. The areas I had initially circled were in reality not the only injuries but only the most extreme of the injuries. This realization was destructive.

My life had been on hold by the more severe injuries for so long that as my combined chiropractic treatments, acupuncture sessions, massage therapies, Pilates classes, and physical therapies slowly tested me, I was able to more clearly determine what I could no longer do. This was when I would kneel to pick up a grocery bag from the floor and realize how horribly awful and painful it was. This was when my physical therapist realized it was unsafe for me to warm up on an exercise bike due to my femoral nerve and other injuries. The warm-up was unbearable and impossible, and it was removed by my therapist. I no longer had any warm-ups, including walking on the treadmill.

In no way do I fault my physical therapist at Location 3, because I think she was great. From her experience, I would never run again. This was devastating and I refused to listen to her. I had built a wall so high that nothing and nobody's words could penetrate. I lived in an alternate world with an alternate reality. In my little world of hope and hard work and innovation, miracles do come true. It had to work. This was my body and my life, and I was not going to give up and adopt a new lifestyle and accept a broken, disabled body. There had to be more. I kept striving, but the pain and trauma and emotional toll was taking me over. I needed a strong support group even more.

When I would eagerly mention kettlebells, my hopes would be dashed again. "I don't think you will ever be able to do kettlebells again," said my physical therapist. This was the stage at which I started to accept my new truth about what body I had left after the semi-truck had ripped it to shreds. My body and brain were trying to reconcile my new reality. This moment was pivotal but also disastrous mentally. It was here at my third physical therapist when I began struggling to get out of bed to go to physical therapy. Physical therapy was no longer fun, and I'd given up

ENERGY, RESEARCH, AND INTELLECT

hope in it. Physical therapy was grueling and painful and it caused more doubts.

Summoning a will and strength beyond my human body's desire, my physical therapy and recovery journey became one of guttural screams, yells, and sobs as I tried to get muscles to activate. I made sounds I'd never made before in my life. I sounded like an animal. I had to rebuild atrophied muscle. I had to reconnect muscle to the brain so the muscle could figure out how to work properly again. I had to work through trauma barriers. Processing the trauma became the most exhausting part of the therapy. It's not a release. It doesn't release endorphins, like laughing. It feels like pulling cells out of your body and being assaulted.

Trauma becomes a part of us. It is part of our cells and our nerves. It is not mental. It's very physical. Our bodies carry the trauma. Trauma is a memory. Trauma is the body crying, the nerves remembering, and the cells holding toxins. When the brain is unconscious, the nerves are still awake. The whole brain is not unconscious. It is still fighting to keep the human alive, and it remembers what the human does not. The brain and nerve memory will eventually tell their story.

My old saying is memories are simply energy. When Einstein died, his memories, which were energy, transformed to another energy form and became stored energy. Then, people were born and absorbed his energy, or memories. Sometimes, his memories ended up in their brain, or other times their arms. When it ended up in their brain, then they have some of Einstein's memory in their brain. They are really smart. I believe this is human evolution. This is why people become smarter, faster as each generation is born. We have previous generations' memories already in our brains for easier recall and to stimulate our nerves and muscles. Energy just evolves. After the tractor-trailer, my nerves, my cells, and my brain were transformed to now store trauma memories. Unfortunately, when I die, that negative energy, trauma, exists and will remain.

To attempt to heal my body, my team ended up using a less-is-more mentality. In hindsight, traditional physical therapy was not working because it was progressing too quickly and started at a level too elevated for my injuries. Initially, I met physical therapy with my normal "can do" attitude. However, it progressed backward once the extent of my injuries was accepted, resulting in me becoming disheartened. It was really traumatizing. I had never gone backward in physical therapy. Unfortunately, physical therapy became a mix of failures and pain, which resulted in me developing trauma to physical therapy.

While physical therapy was focused on hour-long sessions, my chiropractors were focused on the less-is-more. Dr. Murphy believes we are a busy society. It was best to do some kind of exercise instead of nothing. While he applied it to all patients, it worked extremely well for me. I had been accustomed to working out 7-8 hours a week prior to the accident at 1-2 hours on exercise days. This was when I was not marathon training. Post-accident, 30 minutes of physical therapy was too much. This didn't even include cardio. I was struggling to maintain my jobs, eat, and make it to appointments. I was falling apart. Reducing the pressure and stress by telling me it was fine to not do the full repetitions and I did not have to do my physical therapy exercises every day really helped me. I was being put under too much stress. In addition, it also helped by not causing inflammation.

Active Edge's philosophy for healing was a 10 Degree Strategy. It involved only doing 10 degrees more each day for slowly building to doing the full exercise. This plan helped me even more. At Active Edge, they realized just how debilitated my body was and how exercise was taxing my brain. I was becoming too stressed with therapy. I could not do the therapy exercises. I was tired of the pain, disappointment, failures, and setbacks. Establishing 10 degrees and "do what you can" told me I could settle but still do my exercises as best I could without criticism that I was a failure.

I was finally healing.

I also learned nerves remember trauma. Nerves are used every second of the day. For example, nerves are connected to the senses so we can hear

ENERGY, RESEARCH, AND INTELLECT

and see. This is why healing the brain is so slow. Removal of the "senses" is almost necessary to heal. This is why I believe physical therapy needs to be revamped for people with brain injuries and trauma. If a person was in a motor vehicle accident, then even driving to physical therapy can overstimulate the nerves, exhausting the person. Trauma is a lot for the nerves. Doing a full physical therapy session that lasted an hour instead of approaching things from a 10-degree pace with a 15-minute or 30-minute therapy session was likely part of the issue due to the pre-existing trauma and fatigue I had just from the drive to and from therapy.

In 2023, I had a neurologist at the Cleveland Clinic who was very interested in the period of time I had experienced a pain. He was even interested in the time frame of years. He scaled back my rehabilitation to accommodate my nerve pain. To reduce the inflammation and to allow the nerve to relax, I could only do a few exercises to heal the nerve. If it flared, I had to reduce the repetitions of the exercises. I had to rest for days to let soreness or sensation disappear. My doctor clearly explained that the goal was to let the nerve relax and to keep the exercises to a minimum. In comparison, physical therapists usually assigned a significant amount of repetitions. His recommendation matched what I was currently doing with my chiropractic team since I had switched from physical therapists.

Not only was chiropractic and functional medicine pivotal to my healing, but it had to be combined with reducing the workload and stress load that I had endured from traditional physical therapy. Since I was on self-pay, I could move at the slower pace that I needed to heal. To continue finding ways to alleviate my pain, I switched to the Cleveland Clinic for issues that had to be resolved with medicines when my local medical physicians were no longer sufficient. This approach ultimately not only allowed my body to self-heal, but also aided in getting me off of some medications ill-suited for my pain sources while getting me on medications best suited for my medical conditions. The Cleveland Clinic correctly diagnosed multiple sources of pain from the tractor-trailer accident.

PAIN WITH POISE

ACCEPTING MY NEW REALITY

In 2019, Dr. Murphy at MCPC began the process of showing me how doing less was more healing. This was counter to my physical therapy sessions at Location 2, which had followed traditional physical therapy methods while attempting to rehab my neck injury. The hour-long sessions and sets of at-home exercises had caused more pain and increased the inflammation. Dr. Murphy paused my rehab when I arrived at MCPC after quitting rehab at Location 2 to allow the inflammation to reduce. After a few weeks, he restarted my rehab with his "less is more" policy. He assigned 1-2 exercises, stopped focusing on only one injured body region—my neck—and focused on rebuilding my whole body while eliminating inflammation.

This also provided time for me to focus on extracurricular activities such as work, family, and maintaining chores. I had a lot of things to juggle, and I couldn't give up the rest of my life for physical therapy. This helped my mental health and eased the pain. The severe pain I was experiencing in other physical rehabilitation sessions began diminishing.

Cardiovascular exercise was limited to walking and ellipticals at the gym. I would like to say the elliptical was a healthy option, but it also caused pain. I was not able to ride the stationary bike due to my back injury and femoral nerve, so I was limited to a treadmill and elliptical. Both the elliptical and walking on the treadmill hurt. So, I chose the option that hurt the least, which was the elliptical. My list of activities that I was unable to do was still growing.

I was encountering extreme fascia shifts after physical therapy sessions at Location 2, after chiropractic adjustments, and after my first few acupuncture appointments. Extreme fascia shifts can cause a person to pass out, feel light-headed, or feel like a wave is moving across the body. My body needed time to adjust after physical therapy and chiropractic adjustments as well. It wasn't a quick trip to the doctor where my body needed no rest or healing time. In hindsight, I think the workload

ENERGY, RESEARCH, AND INTELLECT

assigned in physical therapy was not allowing my body time to heal. Dr. Murphy started my body on the road to healing with his new approach in my rehabilitation.

Dr. Murphy also educated me on how muscle imbalances would occur due to injured muscles. Even doing physical therapy exercises that were too advanced for my injury were exacerbating those imbalances. I was compensating in how I moved in an attempt to live each day while working, doing chores, etc. These created additional muscle imbalances. In fact, I believed I would have an altered muscle movement forever. I didn't believe I would ever be able to overcome my injuries, since I had leg pain that doctors and therapy were not fixing.

Dr. Murphy got me to start thinking about my injury. He was cautioning me against a 4-mile race I had decided to do in the fall of 2019. I wanted to do the race as a walk for my mental health because I felt like all my dreams, goals, and life were slipping through my fingers. If I could do a race, even as a walk, I could be part of a bigger team and still maintain the mindset that sustained me. While I did do the race and only walked it, he was right. He rehabbed me for weeks afterward even though I had trained to do it. My body was too dysfunctional to walk long distances yet.

Along with my physical therapist at Location 3, Dr. Murphy strongly cautioned me against participating in a particular type of STOTT PILATES**[2] class. The class used mainly a Reformer Apparatus*[*], which offered controlled and gentle movement, instead of a mat. In the fall of 2019, I decided to try this class at the advice of the gym's salesman. I had joined the gym to gain access to equipment I needed to continue my rehabilitation. Anything that may assist in rebalancing my muscles, recover flexibility, and potentially restore my core while being a safe supplement to physical therapy[3] fit my rehabilitation, or so I thought.

However, I had to modify every routine due to pain. I continued attending classes with my instructor's fervent guidance and oversight. However, the COVID-19 lockdown ended our sessions. Then, when I had successful rehabilitation at Active Edge, I realized why I should've waited to participate in these classes. I had fundamental issues that needed to be resolved with precise physical rehabilitation. Simply put, I was too injured to start the class.

However, the sessions allowed me to participate in a group class and let me make friends, which really helped my mental health. Breathing using the diaphragm was our foundation, even though my fascia damage prevented proper breathing. I learned about the vagus nerve. I fell in love with the classes. I believe when my body is ready, these classes will be an excellent opportunity for me to continue improving my strength, flexibility, and health.

At the same time, I was trying to integrate yoga into my recovery. Before the accident, I had considered becoming a yoga instructor. And now, I could not do yoga at all. I tried to do a Warrior III pose for Dr. Murphy to show him something, and he jumped and came running and yelling like I was touching a hot stove. So, I stopped. That was when I learned that it was an unsafe exercise for my back injury.

I had a problem accepting that I was no longer living with a healthy body. I was struggling to relate to and understand my own body. Dr. Murphy opened my brain to the reality of my injury. Acceptance of reality was beginning. This is why it is very important to work with one's medical team when performing any exercise. This is why I began taking every exercise to my therapist for review that I found online.

UNRAVELING THE CONCUSSION

When I told the BWC neurologist, "I think I'm having daily migraines," he told me that was impossible. When I told the Cleveland Clinic neurologist, "I think I'm having daily migraines," he began treatment for my daily migraines. After two years of regulating my migraines at the Cleveland Clinic, I was able to say my pain was improving, and I was

ENERGY, RESEARCH, AND INTELLECT

beginning to feel my old self return. I also noticed changes like my personality beginning to return as well. Turns out, I've been diagnosed with at least two different types of migraines, and they do happen at the same time. Patients really do know more than their doctors sometimes. This is why it's important to recognize one's sixth sense.

A common idea in society is that a concussion heals. I consider it a form of lasting structure alteration, like a scar tissue, because the neuron is injured. For example, while the brain is not bleeding, the neuron is "bruised" or "torn." The neurons are unable to quickly relay information. Even once this is repaired, which can take a very long time, it does not guarantee the neural network will respond in the same way. The brain and body didn't purge themselves of the damaged neurons by killing them. The neurons are dysfunctional. The neural network is likely behaving at a different energy function (See: *The Neural Network*). For this reason, if a person sustains another concussion, research shows it may take longer to heal.

Research shows concussions are also associated with residual head pain. I have head pain, and all of my neurologists have informed me that concussions are known for head pain. The head pain may worsen, linger, and may never go away. Eventually, if a person sustains more and more concussions or even worse head injuries, the person will suffer greatly. If a concussion actually healed completely, it would leave no trace of ever existing in the beginning. There would be no headaches or migraines. Therefore, another head injury would not require a longer healing period.

Think of a sprained ankle. In a way, it's never recovered because it will always have scar tissue within the ligaments. People will often call it the "weaker" ankle. It is more likely to get re-sprained as well. The ligament may become more damaged and the sprain may be of a different grade. I consider the lasting effects of a concussion very similar to those of a sprained ankle. This is why I am a strong advocate for the idea that a concussion leaves lasting alterations and may even promote an environment where concussions are more likely to occur for life. This does not mean the same neuron is damaged in each concussion, or that the same number of neurons are damaged in later concussions. Each concussion is unique. There are billions of neurons in the brain.[4] When people treat the brain like a physical body part, and then begin to treat it like a well-known injury, maybe we will begin to appreciate it more so we can better treat it.

My chiropractors at Active Edge assisted my concussion healing. They introduced me to cranial adjustments. The skull consists of cranial bones which breathe, or have a vibration, even though they are sutured and do not move. Since the cranial bones are designed to breathe, they will react negatively and become irritated when they are hindered. Examples that could hinder their function are when fascia or muscles connected to the cranial bones are overly tight. Dr. Craner highlighted that the cranial bones are connected to all of our fascia chains in some manner. Therefore, fascia chains extending even from the toes are able to affect the cranial bones.

Having my cranial bones adjusted was really painful. However, I always felt better afterward. One reason the cranial bones needed to be adjusted was to help alleviate the stress the cranial nerves were experiencing. Any time the body is under stress, there is inflammation. When there is inflammation, it is harder for the body to heal. As Dr. Craner says, "A stressed state is a diseased state." Nobody wants to live diseased. To aid the nerves in healing, the cranial bones needed to be released. Therefore, I would have adjustments in my mouth, where necessary. This helped ease inflammation of my nerves.

Coincidentally, immediately after the accident, my mouth was full of blisters. I thought these blisters were from glass cuts. I couldn't comprehend why I had so many sores in my mouth—months and years later. I thought I was so sick my body was not healing well. I still had these painful mouth sores in 2020. Turns out, my cranial joints were so restricted my mouth was covered in bumps. Needless to say, the cranial adjustments

ENERGY, RESEARCH, AND INTELLECT

also helped ease my mouth pain. I got my mouth health back. After I began seeking treatment at Active Edge and received cranial adjustments, the really painful sores never returned.

When Dr. Craner heard about all the migraine medications I was prescribed, she began dry needling. Dry needling worked well for my migraines, and my Cleveland Clinic neurologist was very pleased with the results. Combined with my migraine medications, continued chiropractic treatments, and dry needling, I began feeling a lot better.

I have improved function now, and I have more days where I can see clearly and more days where I am able to decipher that I am having a migraine. I still take daily migraine medications, and my neurologist would like to maximize my dosage. However, because I have so many cognitive side effects from the medications, I have refused. I can barely survive the cognitive side effects. I also take prescription migraine medications for when I feel a migraine occurring. For non-migraine headaches, I take OTC migraine medications. As horrible as this sounds, this is a vast improvement from 2020.

My memory recall was strange at times. During casual conversation, my memories felt like they were coming from a black hole. The memory was associated with an abnormal reaction or sensation. For example, my mom recalled a time I vomited vegetable soup on the carpet as a kid. This was a common joke in the family. However, I had no memory of this event after the accident. I became very sick after she mentioned it. The moment my mom mentioned the vomit episode, my brain did not have just an unpleasant memory, but an overwhelming disgusting sensation that overtook me. It caused me pain and discomfort. Because I liked vegetable soup after the accident, I was really annoyed. I can only imagine it was a neural network connection that was damaged. Sometimes, the memory connection is unpleasant, and I describe it as a zapping sensation. Sometimes, the memory may be something I would not want to recall, so I scream and try to stop it. For this reason, I don't like talking to people about my past. I am unable to handle the unpleasant reactions.

PAIN WITH POISE

My neurologists continue to diagnose my head pain. My new neurological physician assistant diagnosed me with idiopathic stabbing headaches in 2023. I thought these were nerve issues. They were so sharp and stabbing. Yet, when I told her about them and another concern I had, she said the pain sounded like these headaches. Unfortunately, there was nothing we could do for them. What she did confirm was I could have several of these severely painful attacks several times a day. They can feel like a stabbing ice pick. She stated this occurrence of headaches and migraines I was experiencing is common after a concussion.

My chiropractor, just like me, wants to eradicate all of my head pain. She's had excellent success with other concussion patients, so we can only hope. The future is always full of hope. For now, I will continue to focus on ways to heal my brain by easing the pain.

15.
DIET AND NUTRITION

I grew up in a family where my mom made everything from scratch and focused on balanced meals. However, I went off to college and ate like all college kids. By graduate school, I had developed gastroesophageal reflux disease (GERDs). I thought I ate relatively healthy and was maintaining a healthy lifestyle. I had fruits and veggies every day. I also exercised daily. However, that was not enough. My second year of enduring GERDs, I revamped my lifestyle and diet. I cut out sugar. I cut out snacking. I focused on portion control. I focused on lean meats, fruits, and veggies. As such, I was able to go off all the antacids and proton-pump inhibitors. Because I forever changed my lifestyle, I never needed to go back on antacids.

During my new journey of health and wellness, I discovered yoga. I did yoga every day before bed. During this time, I exercised in the morning, went to school and did research, came home to exercise, went back to school to do more research, and came home to do yoga before bed. This was my life and I loved it. I also lost so much weight I became the smallest I had ever been as an adult. I weighed a fit 126 pounds.

I also developed a new philosophy about food. I believed food improved one's well-being. I cooked my meals from scratch, ate every two hours, focused on fruits and veggies, made sure to get my protein, and ate healthy carbs like brown rice, whole wheat pasta, and whole wheat bread. I had a regular exercise schedule of runs, a weekly dance lesson, and other cross-training activities. The day I was hit by an 18-wheeler, I was 135 pounds and wore size 6 skinny pants.

PAIN WITH POISE

When I started my new healthy lifestyle in graduate school, I said I would never go back. The accident recovery caused me to slide. I was experiencing a lot of pain and trauma. I was under an extreme amount of stress. Because I couldn't continue my normal exercise routines or daily routines, I had a reduction in burned calories. However, I didn't adjust for this calorie reduction. I wasn't even considering I was eating more than I was living. I was just trying to survive.

I struggled to menu plan. I ran into difficulties with cooking and could no longer sustain my cooking routine. My regular meals were too complicated to make. They required too much energy to make. I no longer had passion to make the meal. I began relying on quick and easy meals that I could toss in the microwave or oven. I also no longer had a planned eating schedule. I began comfort eating, even if that meant buying milkshakes. I learned this eased the pain in my head. I don't know if this was because it really eased the pain in my head due to some nutritional deficit or if it was from something else. I really didn't care. It just gave me some relief.

I ate just to curb the nausea, because I had a life where I lived nauseated from pain. I was so nauseated I didn't even realize I was nauseated. I was in so much pain there would be days I could not drink hot tea. I loved tea. Before the accident, I used to drink it every night before bed. I began this daily ritual in graduate school to eliminate late night eating. The semi-trailer truck stopped this habit. I was in so much pain and I was so nauseated that I was not able to drink a sip of tea. In fact, I didn't even want to drink water.

By 2019, I finally realized my nausea was a real issue. I was cognitively exhausted. My brain couldn't process anything else, including digesting food. I started eating chicken broth. When I tried to eat other foods, it would upset my stomach. I was tired of feeling sick. I changed my eating and drinking habits. Crackers, chicken broth, and ginger ale became my new foods and beverages.

DIET AND NUTRITION

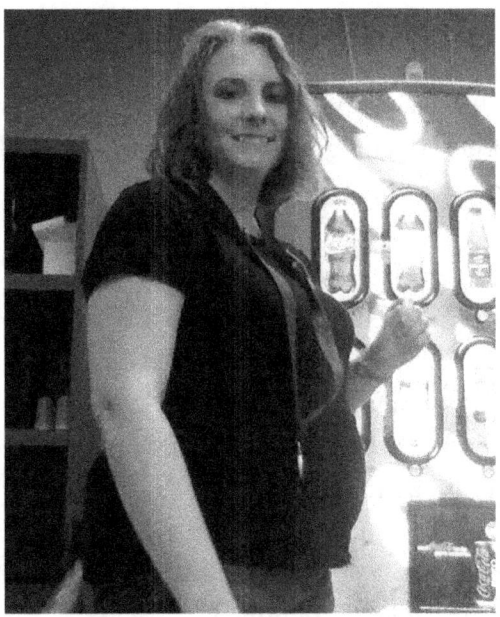

My body after the tractor-trailer accident.

Not only did I buy ginger ale, but I started buying lemon-lime soda to help with the nausea. This was monumental. I stopped drinking soda in undergraduate school and I never went back. However, I finally caved and began drinking a liter a day of ginger ale or lemon-lime soda. My healthy lifestyle ceased. In 2021, I finally stopped drinking soda to switch back to water and tea. However, water was not the same invigorating, fresh taste as it was before the accident. Maybe this was due to nerve irritability or nerve damage in my face affecting my taste buds or olfactory nerves. Maybe it was related to my concussion or just trauma. Maybe it was just because of nausea from pain.

As I had almost been killed, I also decided I should enjoy my life. Why should I not eat sweets? My thought process was, "I could say no to that brownie covered in caramel sauce and walk out the door and be hit by a semi-truck and be six feet under the ground and never see another brownie." Therefore, I decided to eat the brownie.

PAIN WITH POISE

All of this added up to me reaching a lifetime peak weight of 170 pounds within six months of the accident. Going from a fit 135 pounds to an injured 170 pounds on a petite frame was, in a way, catastrophic. I was really concerned and upset about it. I knew the added weight was not helping my recovery or my long-term health. I knew how it was increasing my health risks for diseases like cancer and diabetes. It was also not helping my joints, which had taken a severe beating in the tractor-trailer.

In addition, I noticed my body carried the weight gain differently than it normally did. I had been 160 pounds previously in my life, but it had been a fit 160 pounds. This time, my stomach was really extended from the damaged fascia and core muscles. For the first time in my life, some people were asking for my due date. People thought I was pregnant. The core instability combined with the weight gain made it look like I was pregnant. It was horrendous. None of my clothes fit unless they were yoga pants and sweatshirts. I was slumming it.

In January 2020, I started a diet. I counted calories and input my exercise calories. I allowed sweets in moderation—I may have allowed three pieces of chocolate or two cookies. I successfully lost 20 pounds until the COVID-19 lockdown was issued in March 2020. Like a lot of society, I began to eat unhealthy during the lockdown. However, I didn't gain that much weight. I could never get back to calorie counting though. By 2023, I was suffering from the side effects of my new medications, struggling from my more tedious job, and avoiding pain at all costs. I gained almost all the weight back.

Dieting was harder after the accident, resulting in increased pain. The nerves would become alive and fiery in my face so I would usually slap myself. In a way, trying to diet was a sadistic process, especially since I was also eating to deal with pain. Self-control increased pain and my exhaustion, because I would have to be more structured, more ordered, and still try to do it while poised. Self-control was against nature.

To tell a person in pain or dealing from a significant trauma to behave

DIET AND NUTRITION

a certain way or critique them was ludicrous simply because of the second law of thermodynamics. The universe tends to disorder. To stay rigid with meals and to fight cravings was painful. I couldn't endure the pain. I instead chose to eat. Dieting and portion control increased stress. I could feel the added stress in my body, and the spasms and pain would increase. While I lost weight, I was in misery. I felt like I was burning alive.

By 2021 and 2022, I was running on sheer willpower. My body was taxed. It was being put on medications and taken off of medications, enduring extreme long-term pain, enduring extreme mental, physical, and emotional tolls, and trying to heal. Somehow, I was trying to survive normal life, too. Even with a not-so-great diet, I was able to resume great bowel health once my core redeveloped after years of rehabilitation. To this day, I have a lot of food aversions. It's really hard to eat healthy now.

Reviewing what I endured during my trauma and healing, I think it's important to prepare those who suffer from extreme health events with nutritional advice. At the very least, doctors should find out what a person's normal diet and nutrition plan is so they can use that to see how a person's lifestyle is altered by their injury. This will aid in determining the extent of the person's injury. I was thankful my doctors never criticized me for my weight gain. A person shouldn't be faced with worsening health in one area while trying to recover from pain and trauma.

As Active Edge focused on functional health, they also suggested supplements and focused on the brain-gut connection. While this was not a major aspect to my recovery, I was also in an environment that kept me educated and aware of nutrition's relationship to my well-being. I would add supplements to my diet that also made water taste better, which helped me drink more water—a definite positive for my health.

16.
THE TRANSITION

It appeared I had been successfully overcoming challenges during my recovery until 2020. I started a new job so I wouldn't stay at home during the COVID lockdown. While I was still in a lot of pain and could barely function, I was definitely trying to do things.

Then, I had a detached retina surgery late 2020, and I became tired. I didn't feel the way I did after surgery like I did before the surgery. My theory was that my body was under so much stress from trying to recover from the tractor-trailer, it was unable to handle the added stress from the surgery. I never rebounded. I also had a complication from my first surgery. I needed a second surgery to fix a macular pucker within six months. The surgery was brutal. I had an even worse recovery. I believe the underlying conditions from my semi-trailer truck injury made my recovery even more difficult.

In 2021, I started taking prescription migraine medications on a daily basis. My brain was feeling better, because it was now in less pain. However, it was about this time that I crashed. I initially lost a couple of pounds as a side effect of the medication, and then everything ceased. My strong drive to work, my perseverance, and my clarity vanished. I suddenly struggled to get out of bed. I made it to work but something felt wrong. I began to complain to people that I felt horrible. It wasn't even a depression. Something just felt bad. This period continued for months. I complained to my managers for months about feeling really, really bad. I felt like a sandbag in my bed. I barely made it out of bed to work. I was continually late to work.

PAIN WITH POISE

During this time, I started dreading even going to my chiropractor. I went from doing Essentrics® every morning to no longer working out. I no longer wanted to do any exercises. I regained 10 pounds. It was like I had no ability to care about what I ate, to understand what I was eating, or how much I ate. Ironically, my migraine medications were working. My pain was decreasing. I did consider that I was finally settling down and healing. My brain was suffering less and less. I considered that my brain was now demanding the rest it needed. I decided I was finally in a phase of healing rest. I don't know if it was my body and brain suddenly saying, "Enough!" But, it finally crashed.

By fall 2021, I really began to deteriorate. I went from working out every day to completely being unable to function by late fall of 2021. I could barely get out of bed. My brain was in a total fog. It wouldn't even function to organize my day. Exercises I used to easily complete I could no longer do. My knees hurt. I didn't even want to eat because food was too hard to eat unless it was sweets. I was walking into work and complaining every day. I kept saying, "I don't know what is wrong with me, but I feel awful." I had been coming back from the tractor-trailer accident at Active Edge, and now it felt like my recovery had reached its end. My body had reached its limit. There was a permanent disability that my body could not overcome. It felt like the other medical practitioners had been right—I was never coming back. I had established an unrealistic dream for reclaiming my life.

Then, I endured a very stressful holiday season at Kohl's. I didn't even want to celebrate Christmas even though I loved Christmas. In comparison, I decorated the year of my accident using modified decorations. I found my small pre-decorated Christmas tree and set it up. I had even creatively wrapped gifts even though I couldn't move to wrap gifts. Christmas 2022 I didn't want to wrap presents or decorate.

It felt like I had to consciously use my brain to move each part of my body. The brain-body connection was *that* exhausting and abnormal. My

THE TRANSITION

chiropractor finally tested me for adrenal fatigue. I took the recommended supplements. Over time, I noticed improvements in my brain, and I was able to exercise more. I started to have an appetite for healthy foods and no longer craved sweets. I could monitor and control my eating. My knees stopped hurting. I no longer had to think to wake up my brain. However, I still wasn't completely back. I was struggling to return to what I had been in 2021.

Ironically during this time, I began to notice essential changes to my body. Everything I had been fighting so hard to get to work was suddenly fitting back together. I was applying the breathing techniques. I was sleeping and resting. It was like my body suddenly got what it needed to heal.

Was this a peaceful transition? Did I find my inner me and discover why this happened to me? No, this was probably my angriest phase. I was starting to come to terms with how, four years later, my life was looking so different than I had planned. I was having to accept how different I'd become. I was having to wonder if the person of 2018 was gone forever. There was still no husband and definitely no boyfriend. In fact, I was more hateful about men than before. The journey showed me how society hates. I had been introduced to a world that was foreign to me and was having to wonder if that was the real world—cynical, selfish, and shallow. I had lost hope.

Yet, I held onto things that had once inspired me. I remembered a YouTube video of a military veteran by the name of Arthur, who had overcome a great disability using yoga.[1] He had been told by his doctors he would never walk again without assistance. Yet, he was able to heal his body with yoga. While I was not finding it possible to do the same, I kept going. There was still determination even if I was no longer able to feel hope. I guess it was like God. I can't see, feel, or smell God, but I knew he was there. This time, I could not feel hope like I normally did, yet I was still living with hope.

As 2022 continued, I did continue to notice subtle changes with my brain. I stayed on my migraine medications and my neurologist continued to increase the dosage. The one benefit of eliminating or easing chronic

PAIN WITH POISE

pain was body parts could heal. I started seeing this healing. I said I felt like my personality started to return. Over time, I began to notice other things begin to return. By fall of 2022, I noticed a huge change in my whole body. In fact, some things were beginning to return to pre-accident normal. Other things were still out of whack. Other times, I would be talking to get all the trauma and pain to release and—wham! I would suddenly re-align to be one within myself. I would no longer be struggling with trauma or pain. I would be whole. It was the oddest experience.

For most of 2022, my exercise routine became working at Kohl's and sometimes pulling myself together to do a few exercises once a week. It did not add up to 30 minutes. This was in comparison to when I was doing two hours several days a week during physical therapy up through 2020. Regardless, I healed. After my strange crash in late 2022, I started the slow process of running.

17.
JUSTICE

While I had emerged thankful from my car, the injustices and hate throughout the years slowly destroyed me. Bit by bit, I no longer recognized myself. I began to live in anger and fear, because I was treated badly. Even though I wanted justice, I was denied. In the meantime, door after door after door slammed in my face. The glorious gift of being given more time on Earth started to feel like a curse.

As the negative influences overcame the positive influences, I tried to carve out a hole to find some outlet to hold onto hope. My hope was to overcome. My hope was not to destroy. My hope was to free. My hope was not to oppress. My hope was to inform. My hope was not to erase.

After the accident, I had several goals. I wanted to run again. I wanted to be independent and resume my professional career. I wanted to pursue normal life stuff, such as dating, vacations, and hanging out with friends. I was going to find the miracle to get better. I began analyzing my body to find that miracle.

I fought the COVID lockdown. I found a medical team that listened to me, uniquely treated my pain, and rehabbed me using functional medicine and innovative techniques. I have a professional career. I am independent. My professional career is not what I was expecting. I am still struggling to have a steady career that I enjoy. Cracking the professional mold is very challenging. There are too many variables. As for pursing normal life, I don't date. I ceased hanging out with some groups, because they didn't understand my health situation.

PAIN WITH POISE

As I contemplated how to react to people breaking me down, I considered poise. I always maintained my composure, even when I had failed my first-year physical chemistry oral exam at The Ohio State University. I maintained my poise with smiles when I ran in pain. However, the pain from this journey was too much. The pain seeped through the cracks. The pain took over. The pain triggered curse words and outbursts. The more people stressed me, the more my body succumbed to the pain. Yet, people expected me to maintain my poise.

People wanted me to say I was beyond blessed by being given life. In reality, I was in horror meeting a version of me I never knew could exist. I was facing an identity crisis. I was realizing how wrong I had been about others who went through their own traumas. While my world turned upside down, I came to know being superhuman. I had superhuman strength. I saw things from surreal perspectives. I understood life as if God himself walked with me. Yet, when walking with God, it was like I faced all of evil. I loved God. Yet, I also hated God. I wondered why God hated me. Why had God not wanted me to stay with Him in heaven? While I faced this quandary, I strangely felt sane because the world I was re-entering was so insane.

I saw quotes about leadership on the walls of my doctors' offices and left with a sour taste in my mouth. What did they know about leadership as they laughed at my pain? As they closed doors that increased my stress and pain? As they judged and stereotyped? I saw quotes about integrity and ethics at professional environments in which I was air slapped and people in pain were mocked. I saw quotes about inclusion where the pain-ridden were prevented access to pain management resources during COVID. Leadership, on planet Earth, is used primarily for fame. It's used for money. It's used for notoriety. It's used to mislead. So, I held on to God.

Through this journey, my soul, heart, and mind faced their biggest breaks. The cruelties I endured were endless. Justice didn't exist. I faced a reality that included fighting the rest of my life to maintain a job, to live without pain, and to function. I faced a reality of conforming to a

JUSTICE

world in which I no longer belonged or wanted to belong. So, I fought to change perspectives. I had dreams I was still endlessly fighting to achieve, which would require overcoming monumental obstacles. I had proven many wrong, yet I had so many to still prove wrong. I wanted to live in an accepting world, where the disabled and non-disabled succeed as one. In the meantime, I now knew pain with poise.

PART 2
REHABILITATION IN DETAIL

Once you put human life in human hands,
you have started on a slippery slope that knows no boundaries.
—Dr. Leon Kass[1]

NOTE FROM THE AUTHOR

The exercises I performed during my recovery are from the many years of exercises assigned by physical therapists, chiropractors, and movement coaches during my rehabilitation, as well as what I found when I researched exercises online. The selection of exercises I chose for this book are those that I personally consider the most useful for healing. Based on my experience, these exercises have the potential to heal neurological or high-impact injuries more quickly by treating the source of the issue in a more precise, controlled manner. This decreases stress while easing pain and inflammation in the patient.

18.
VISUALIZATION & PHYSICAL REHABILITATION

As the days and months passed, I tried to do more physically so I could regain a normal life. This was when I realized how much was actually wrong with my body. As physical rehabilitation proceeded at Location 2, it didn't progress as expected. I became concerned, and I decided to dramatically shake things up. I had successfully completed rehabilitation in the past. Most notably, I had used chiropractors as part of my rehabilitation. When I made my first sudden rehabilitation change in 2019, I went to a chiropractor.

After a period of rest from traditional physical therapy, in the first half of 2019, I returned to physical therapy. My new family doctor wanted me to see a physical therapist for my lower body injuries, because those had been ignored so far in my recovery. I wanted to find a physical therapist who gave me total control, in case this doctor and I had a conflict in how to care for my body as well. Since this physical therapist didn't require a doctor referral, the match was ideal.

By summer 2019, I was at Location 3. The physical therapist suggested I was suffering from neurological weakness of my lower extremities. Neurological weakness sucked. No matter how much force or effort was applied, nothing happened. In January 2020, I encountered my most alarming episode of neurological weakness. I had one step to take into the house from my garage. This particular day, I could not go up and into my house. I had to use so much exertion to power myself into the house, I was in disbelief. I was experiencing neurological weakness. I almost didn't make it inside.

PAIN WITH POISE

At Location 3, my physical therapist explained I was having to retrain the muscle of my lower body to work with my brain. Normally, neurons relay information to muscles, which result in the muscles moving in the desired coordination.

This activation of muscles is called muscle synergy.[1] Neurological weakness is when these neurons do not communicate the message correctly. In this case, it is much harder to perform a movement than it should be.

This was the first time I considered my injury to be severe. While my doctors never mentioned neurological weakness to me, I knew I had an amazing physical therapist. Since I was having so many issues with my doctors understanding and diagnosing my injuries, I decided this was a more accurate assessment of my injuries. It was no longer about an injured muscle needing to heal. Now, I had to consider that there was a disconnect between my brain and muscle somewhere along the neural network. While I didn't have spinal cord damage, something was not connecting correctly.

VISUALIZATION

I began practicing visualization to help my brain and neurons. Visualization provided the opportunity for my brain to envision a perfect form to ease my body into the correct form. It encouraged the muscles that were not working properly to start coordinating together by mimicking what I was telling them to do. Using visualizing was not new to me. Before the accident, I had used it on training runs to train my body and to keep proper form when fatigue would hit on long runs. I searched online for how anatomy looked. I began visualizing my anatomy and how it should move.

To activate my numb glutes, I visualized my glute muscle like it was an anatomy diagram in a textbook. To do a left front leg lift, I would visualize the abdominal muscles next to my left pelvis with ligaments and tendons. It was an inaccurate image, but with enough visualization and

VISUALIZATION & PHYSICAL REHABILITATION

thought, it worked. It took years of rehabilitation and visualization to be able to do the movement, a single leg lift, but I believe it was the combination that resulted in the successful reconnection of brain and muscle to allow the movement.

Unfortunately, visualizing didn't magically solve my rehabilitation issues. I actually became exhausted. This was contrary to what happened to me when I practiced visualization as a runner. As a runner, visualization was a way to trick my brain into giving me a positive lift. I actually used visualization strategies to keep going during mental ruts during long runs, like marathons. Therefore, I mentally and physically trained myself on all runs to be a winner using visualization. Post-accident, however, this mental exercise tasked my pain-ridden, trauma-tolled, and concussed brain so much that my brain eventually exhausted before my body. My brain exhausted quickly in physical therapy. Then, after days, weeks, and months of visualizing, my brain began struggling to visualize.

When I had sustained a concussion years prior, my neurologist in Cleveland, Ohio, had suggested cognitive rehabilitation. I went to cognitive therapy at OhioHealth Neurological Rehabilitation in Columbus, Ohio, to retrain my brain for small tasks, such as planning and memory recall. At therapy, I learned that if I began to tire and felt a headache begin, we were to stop the session for the day. Sometimes our sessions lasted 10 minutes. They never lasted longer than 15 minutes. We only did one session a week. We did sessions with the lights off. My occupational therapist told me that the moment pain began, healing ended. This enlightened me to how damaging pain was to the brain. It showed me how quickly external and internal stimulation could overwork the brain and result in pain (See: *The Neural Network* in Chapter 27). Pain was a sign of something going wrong in the brain.

This made me start thinking about what I was being subjected to during my physical rehabilitation. A typical physical therapy session lasted about an hour. The brain had to work to heal the broken and injured body parts in a physical therapy session. This was in addition to what my brain

PAIN WITH POISE

was trying to do at rest, such as at home or even sleeping. The brain was not disconnected in physical therapy. This got me thinking. Was a standard physical therapy session asking too much of brain-injured patients? Should physical therapy sessions be shortened because physical therapy was also exercising, which taxed the injured brain? Should at-home physical therapy assignments be decreased for those recovering from brain injuries? Limiting the scope of this idea to only brain-injured patients was too extreme, though. I believed it should include people who suffered traumatic injuries, which included emotional and cognitive injuries.

I was also dealing with physical pain, which refused to go away. As my pain persisted for years, it began to tax my brain even more. This was when I learned the cognitive toll that pain had on a person. Cognition is the process of establishing an information database in the brain so a human can move, converse, and evolve. Some examples of cognitive processes are attention span, language skills, reasoning, sensation, external perception, and movement.[2] My brain had initially struggled from my concussion. Years later, my brain was struggling from the added toll of chronic pain. This domino effect was greatly affecting my cognitive health. This was when I began my new awareness of pain and the appreciation of managing pain. To heal, I had to account for brain strain from all contributing factors draining my cognitive energies.

To visualize through pain meant I was visualizing all day. That process wore me out. Instead, I tried to stay active and busy with tasks. I tried to stay connected with people. I tried to stay distracted so I was not having to make my brain trick itself all day long that I was not in pain. However, to stay busy with tasks required a significant amount of physical and mental exertion for the state of health I had. I wore out. I had an injured body. I had pain. I had dysfunctional neural networks in my brain. While trying to outdo the pain, I was becoming exhausted. My ability to stay distracted from the pain or with visualizing in order to heal started growing shorter and shorter over the years.

VISUALIZATION & PHYSICAL REHABILITATION

One major benefit to visualization during physical rehabilitation was preventing overcompensation of the wrong muscles. This was vital to healing, because I had to break the bad habit of using other muscles that were stronger and had begun compensating for my weaker, dysfunctional muscles. For this reason, visualizing was essential to isolating the correct muscle in order to retrain the muscle and brain connection. Sometimes, I felt rushed through exercises with physical therapists. At home, I learned the art of breaks between each exercise to visualize and reposition. If I went too fast, I would engage the wrong muscles. This would result in overcompensating with the stronger muscle and using an incorrect muscle synergy.

The process proceeded via the following steps.

1. Rest after a rep of performing the exercise.
2. Take assessment of my body.
3. Disengage body parts that were trying to lock.
4. Visualize the body parts in the exercise moving.
5. Perform the exercise again.

In reality, I was repositioning after each rep. Physical therapy became more mental than physical. For me to isolate the correct muscle required so much brain power that my brain became exhausted. As my brain burned out, I was left unable to do the exercise correctly. Then, a bawling, negative person remained. Visualization began to drive my brain into exhaustion.

As a result, I began skipping physical therapy sessions. I dreaded them. They hurt, and they made me feel bad about myself. I was losing hope. I was tired of being sick and having injuries. I was tired of facing the severity of my injuries. The present was full of little distractions from constant pain, worry, grief, and going to another medical appointment. I was facing medical burnout. Where I used to embrace the medical world as one necessary to get me better, it was now a dreaded part of my life. The medical world was also a place where hope had been replaced with fear. My new reality was that nothing would heal my body.

MINDFULNESS AND THE SOUL

I also practiced visualization for mental health. I tried Holographic Manipulation Therapy® (HMT) at Active Edge. I found this practice interesting. Sometimes, when my memory was strong, I remembered to use the technique at home. However, I had a physical impairment that distracted me during the therapy. Post-therapy, I decided I was stating the wrong emotions. Time and trauma were tainting my perspectives. Finally, as it used visualization during the therapy session, I often struggled to maintain the mental power to do the visualization.

Over the months, I considered trying HMT again or another form of psychotherapy. However, there was something about thinking about events and dissecting them that was just ugly to me. I just wanted to live and move forward. With physical rehabilitation, I had endured constant analysis of myself. I was done. I was burned out. Even though it worked for many people, I decided to live life to the fullest to maintain my mental health.

Part of this living life to the fullest was experiencing the world. I had always loved vacationing. I enjoyed the opportunity to meet strangers. I had always enjoyed traveling for runs, even solo. I loved people. When the accident occurred, this love for people changed. This is why I say I lost my personality soon after the accident. I was needing to stay so positive in such a negative environment that I was emotionally drained. To save myself, I had begun detaching from humans. By 2021, I noticed these changes within myself. I was no longer making eye contact.

It was on a trip to Seabrook Island, South Carolina, in 2022 that I could finally feel God trying to reconnect with me using the universe. I stood on the beach and let the ocean take over my brain. This was a completely different trip than when I went to Seabrook Island three years prior to celebrate

VISUALIZATION & PHYSICAL REHABILITATION

being able to see the beach for the first time after my accident. My 2019 trip was pure joy. That trip was celebrating I was alive and graced with the ability to experience the sand and the ocean after a near-death experience. Now, I was an empty shell feeling nothing but pain. I had endured such an onslaught from medical practitioners, so-called friends turned ghosts, potential boyfriends, and functioning on autopilot in my professional life to survive and get through hell. I visualized what was on the other side of the ocean. My brain began to reset. My heart tried to purge.

Everywhere I went on the island, people smiled, waved, and greeted me. They were not forced greetings, but genuine greetings. They were greetings coming from a place deep within that said, "I like myself and who I am." They were all so friendly and hospitable. They were all full of joy and goals and stories that were trying to fill my empty bucket. And, they were strangers. By my last day there, I finally felt the change. I started feeling a connection to the ocean like I usually do. The trip worked so well that I began scheduling more vacations to relearn the world.

In 2023, my job put together a little game. One option for the game was to perform 30 minutes of meditation. I decided to try meditating. I had tried various styles of mindfulness over the years since the accident and none of it was working. Before the semi-truck, I greatly appreciated the art of mindfulness and regularly practiced it. Mindfulness could be performed in several manners in order for a person to find the therapies to match their personality. Therapies included breathing, acceptance without judgment, focusing and maintaining attention, or even therapeutic exercise, like yoga.[3]

As these practices indicated, mindfulness was great for both the mind and the body, because it utilized the body for centering the mind. As everyone deals with stress, mindfulness could be a great option for balancing a person's stress. Mindfulness was also culturally accepted among all, and could be practiced in a variety of forms, as it was both flexible and adaptable.

I decided to do breathing for my mindfulness therapy. Instead of

PAIN WITH POISE

starting with 30 minutes, I decided to do five-minute intervals to add up to 30 minutes for one day. The first five minutes were awful. My mind traveled everywhere. I was extremely impatient. My mind was so used to multi-tasking. I was trying to plan my next day's relaxing vacation in my head. I kept hearing kids playing in the distance. I would start to think about dinner plans. My mind was jumping everywhere.

No matter how many times I did it, five minutes lasted forever. However, the more I did it, the more I noticed changes and the quieter my brain became. I even started to get into the zone. I tried taking a quick walk around the park between five-minute meditation sessions. This helped calm my mind even more. I decided to add it to my regular routine to see if it helped my brain.

REHABILITATION THERAPIES

Essentrics®

I was introduced to Essentrics® by one of my massage therapists in the fall of 2021. I began following Miranda Esmonde-White, a former ballerina turned healthy aging PBS fitness expert and New York Times bestselling author of the Aging Backwards series on YouTube. She created the science-based Essentrics® Workout—a full body workout that rebalances your body by dynamically stretching and strengthening all your muscles and taking all your joints through their full range of motion. It uses gentle, rotational movements, along with large, full body exercises that will allow you to explore all planes of movement. Essentrics® helps to restore balance and movement in your body, increase flexibility and mobility, and relieve pain and stiffness.

I discovered that their technique has been used by professional athletes including the NHL's Montreal Canadiens and Olympians over the past 25 years. It was amazing for my recovery.

The routine would bring about fatigue while exercising. However,

VISUALIZATION & PHYSICAL REHABILITATION

when I completed my workout, I wasn't exhausted. This contradicted what I experienced with physical therapy sessions. After physical therapy, I had to ice and would want to do nothing for the rest of the day. I started to recognize a huge difference in my body and learned what areas of my body I needed to develop. I highlighted these weaknesses to my chiropractor for additional feedback. Essentrics® became essential to my recovery.

Walking

I trained for the M3S Sports The Ohio State 4-Miler in the fall of 2019. I did this for my mental health. I had reached a low point and decided to register. Again, my physical therapist was concerned and doubtful. My chiropractor likely felt the same way. I was a runner and I registered for races. These races helped me connect and achieve goals with others. This was lacking in my recovery. I did train to walk the race and I still regretted doing the race. I couldn't turn my head left or right the whole walk. I was too restricted. My recovery was horrible. It took months before I felt like I had pre-race. My chiropractor had to fix everything. I ended up returning to only walking one mile for exercise very slowly.

Exercise DVDs

I used to use exercise DVDs, such as Walk Away the Pounds (WAP) with Leslie Sansone, yoga, Pilates, dance, and Billy Blanks Tae Bo for cross-training. In 2019, I decided to try my old WAP exercise DVDs. I could tell something was wrong, because it was brutal to perform the exercises. I couldn't do the arm exercises while I was walking. In addition, walking at the speed they wanted was too hard and painful. Each footfall shot pain up my back and spine. Each attempt to walk faster caused my groin, abdomen, and back to scream.

Walking in place to the DVD routine at my slow pace was depressing. I quit doing them. This was when I realized the warning that appears at the start of exercise DVDs that says "Do not try without consulting with your doctor" actually mattered. It applied to me.

After using the breathing techniques to rebuild my core and Essentrics®, I began to try my exercise DVDs again in 2022. I was able to do my dancing DVDs. I slowly began to incorporate my yoga DVDs as my yoga poses needed a lot of modifications. I was also able to do the WAP DVDs with modifications. For the weights, I started with soup cans. In 2024, I began cautiously performing basic martial arts kicks. I know I will be able to do my Tae Bo DVDs again as well.

Vagus Nerve

One of the most beneficial things I learned in my Pilates class was to reset my vagus nerve. This provided a cleanse that always resulted in a big cry.

The vagus nerve is the main component of the parasympathetic nervous system which controls mood, digestion, immune response, and heart rate.[4] Stimulating the vagus nerve is believed to assist in stress regulation, mood regulation, and assisting with treatment of post-traumatic stress disorder. For me, it resulted in a huge emotional release.

The first time I did it, I was unable to get my right side to reset. I was told to stop and look left. It reset within 5 minutes. Then, I was told to look right again and it reset within 5 minutes. My whole nervous system was really suffering. I can tell the difference today with my improved overall well-being. Now it takes my vagus nerve 5 seconds or less to reset.

Facial Yoga

My face reflected the accident for years after it occurred. I used to naturally smile, and my friend Randy said I had a smile that "lit up the room." The muscles in my face were connected to the muscles in my neck, and all were harmed by the semi-trailer truck As things became more difficult,

VISUALIZATION & PHYSICAL REHABILITATION

the left side of my face became more drawn. The corners of my lips began turning down more and more.

In order for my mouth to form a smile, I had to have very positive thoughts and truly feel positive in the moment. The more pain I was in, the more both sides of my lips would turn down at a harsh angle. I caught myself looking this way in a photo from my 5k.

During a smile, it can feel like pulling against clay to get both of my lips curled upward. When I smile, it's like I can feel the roof of my mouth tugging as I have very tight muscles. It's actually very challenging for me to smile.

In 2023, I Googled "facial yoga." I discovered it was an actual thing. As there are muscles in a person's face, it was not about vanity. It was a necessity. The muscles in my face were tight and likely atrophied. When I do facial yoga, I can feel a difference in my face. I am more prone to smiling.

Acupuncture

Acupuncture is a therapy that uses acupuncture needles placed into acupoints[5] to help the body rebalance naturally. Acupuncture uses meridians, which are lines of energy in the body, to promote health.[6] It is commonly helpful for chronic pain[7] caused by both physical and emotional components.[8]

I had never gone to acupuncture before, and I was extremely nervous. My acupuncturist chose to not use electric stimulation as I was unable to tolerate it. The first few sessions, I experienced an extreme shifting. It was like something within my whole body was moving, including within my head. It was unsettling. In addition, I also experienced dizzy spells for hours. Eventually, these issues went away, and acupuncture became a more tolerable experience.

Massage Therapy

I didn't want foot rubs or back rubs. The pain was too intense. I was numb to foot rubs. I quickly learned to never use massage chairs. My work had one and I paid for it with excruciating back spasms; my muscles and fascia were so destroyed and weakened they were no longer able to handle the pressure. I still do not use a chair massager; I'm part of a very small percentage of people who cannot.

However, my thought was that, in order to get better, I had to release toxins, decrease stress, and do tissue work. I decided to start massage therapy. I went to my longtime massage therapist who had been with me through marathon training. This time though, the massage was almost unbearable to endure. I dreaded lying upside down as strange things would ensue like jerking to full alertness and gasping for air when areas of my back would be touched. Large portions of my massage sessions were focused on my abdomen, which had been destroyed. In addition, I had an area on the left side of my back that felt like it had been injected with asphalt. When the therapist worked on it, the pain surged and I would have difficulty breathing. Depending upon what areas of my back had pressure applied, I would struggle to breathe. Over the course of years, I have learned my reaction was from nerve pain.

Because of the irritated nerves, I have had neurologists advise no longer having massage therapy as a part of my healing plan to allow the nerves to rest and heal. This has proven to be a very frustrating aspect to recovery.

Dry Needling

Dry needling is a therapy where a needle is inserted deeply into a trigger point in the fascia or muscle and left to release a knot or trigger point. This technique can help decrease pain, spasms, and trigger points.[9] I had dry needling in several body parts, but mostly my head, neck, and face.

VISUALIZATION & PHYSICAL REHABILITATION

e-stim

I also used e-stim therapy. Ironically, none of my physical therapists used e-stim. Only my chiropractors used it. e-stim is a therapy where electrical pulses are sent through the skin to stimulate either muscles or nerves to promote healing and reduce pain.[11]

Aromatherapy

As I preferred being as natural as possible in my life and already used essential oils for cleaning—such as tea tree oil—I believed in the benefits of essential oils. In 2018, a friend introduced me to using essential oils for pain relief. I relied heavily on a roll-on to get me through my pain. It worked so well.

Active Edge used essential oils for disinfecting, topical use, and as a room fragrance. Just walking into Active Edge made me feel better. I decided it had to be the essential oils. They had essential oil soap, lotions, and diffusers. They used disinfectants on their tables with essential oils, and this made even painful adjustments tolerable. I really wanted to get started on essential oils at my house. I hoped it would have the same effect on me at home. However, essential oils were really expensive. I couldn't justify paying for them. So I started with just lavender from the retail store. I used it at night when going to bed to try and help me sleep since I was no longer sleeping.

In 2023, I began purchasing essential oils. I searched the Internet for a good quality brand. I chose to splurge on rose essential oil because I learned since the accident that I loved the smell of rose. I find this interesting because I always hated the smell of rose prior to the accident. I also bought ylang ylang, peppermint, orange, lemon, and lavender for my initial basic set. I learned to avoid anything smoky, as that can result in a claustrophobic feeling.

I also learned to be careful with essential oils. Some essential oils do not mix well with medical conditions, such as epilepsy. Therefore, it's necessary to do research into which essential oils I can use and which to avoid.

Cupping Therapy

My massage therapist utilized cupping in my massage therapy. Christina Murphy, DC, also practices cupping at MCPC. I bought my own silicone cupping set to use at home. Cupping is wonderful for releasing fascia. I focus on my neck, shoulders, upper back, and chest.

Pranic Healing

No matter what my team did, I still had issues with my head and neck. I still was in horrific pain. I still felt like something was inside the side of my head. My face was spasming horribly. Then I was introduced to pranic healing. Pranic healing is a type of therapy which uses energy to locate and resolve areas of injury or inflammation. It is founded in quantum physics and self-awareness. The connection between the mind, body, and soul is used to guide the focused mind to become connected to the self during massage therapy. It is a unique therapy for both physical and emotional concerns.[10]

During a session, Sybil Baker, a licensed massage therapist specializing (LMT) in pranic healing, would locate a dysfunctional body area and then begin treating it. She would also inquire about what happened to that area. She would then piece together the puzzle of how the accident may have impacted and damaged my body. She also rebalanced the brain after traumas, such as concussions or post-traumatic stress disorder.

During my recovery, I had developed an annoying issue with my left ear popping and feeling like something was inside, stabbing it. I had complained quite loudly of it. My head was also crooked the majority of the time. I had done lots of stretching and neck exercises, but it was still crooked. Sybil not only immediately noticed this, but during my treatment, I actually noticed how things started to move in the room because of the rotation in my head from a barely imperceptible pressure she applied to my neck and shoulder region. In fact, it was like vertigo. I had to ask if things were really moving. She stated that it was indeed my head. The rest

VISUALIZATION & PHYSICAL REHABILITATION

of the day I felt so much better. I didn't think about taking one migraine med or needing any pain medications. I didn't have one facial spasm.

In addition, she treated my left shoulder. This was the part of my body that the tractor-trailer hit. My car seat had been rotated. My best guess was the semi-trailer truck had hit the edge of my seat so my shoulder had taken a beating. Sybil said it was energetically disconnected, so she worked on it and stated it was twisted. Again, I felt no pain like one may feel in a massage. However, I started feeling twinges on my right side, along my right leg, right arm down to my wrist, and along the right side of my neck. I went home later and did some crunches. To my shock, that area of my body heated up. What she had done worked that well.

19.
THE MIRAGE OF POISE

THE EVOLUTION OF POISE

While society tries hard to consider each individual patient's needs, gaps still remain. Society tries to fill these gaps most often with equality. Equality means giving everybody the same tools to try to achieve the same goal. However, some will not succeed. Instead, equity is far more beneficial at providing each individual person what is necessary to achieve the same goal.

In the equality illustration shown in Figure 1, the three people in pain after sustaining their injuries are provided the same medical tool, a medical bandage, to return to living life after their injury. However, the bandage is not enough for all people to return to living life. This means equality is insufficient to overcome the differences the injury has caused in each person. In comparison, the equity illustration shows different medical tools are provided to each injured person. One person needs a brace, one person needs a crutch, and one person needs a wheelchair and back brace to return to living their lives.

When translated to a disability, one person may have one million things wrong with them compared to another person's two things. Equity means more time off work, more rest, and special rehabilitation must be given to the person who has one million things wrong with them versus the person with only two things. Equity means accepting the reality of one's real disabilities to end compartmentalizing injuries and textbook treating to heal a person.

PAIN WITH POISE

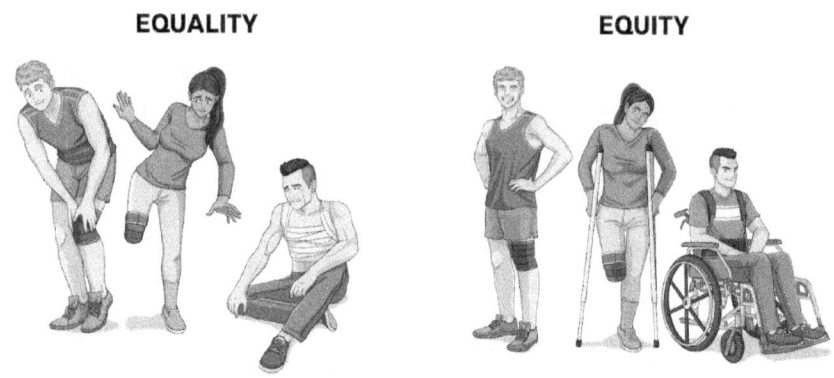

Figure 1. Illustrated by Charis, *Equality and Equity*, Fiverr, March 13, 2024.

After analyzing what worked and what didn't work to heal me, I saw trends and decided they might help others. With this journey toward a more equitable healthcare, POISE emerged. I created POISE as an incremental-based therapy with a focus on rest, which applies visualization and breathing techniques to heal. While POISE was developed to rehab nerves, muscles, and fascia from a high-impact accident, it can be adapted for those with whiplash from any impact, suffering from core instability such as in pregnancy, and for regaining flexibility from back injuries. I created POISE so that others would be able to reclaim their active lifestyle from pain by building strength and decreasing inflammation from injuries ranging from moderate to severe. It relied on trial and error for the program to be a success. Success also relied on rehabilitation application. In addition, as I struggled with relationships during my recovery because I had needs that caused conflict with others, I offer some suggestions on how to take care of sick family and friends.

POISE discourages compartmentalizing body parts for treatment. It encourages considering the patient as a functioning body of joints, muscles, and fascia instead of as unrelated individual parts. The therapist should determine the patient's health and/or injury status using a comprehensive body assessment. The therapist must maintain the mindset that the body works as a whole to heal. The injured body part(s) are attached to a brain, which can be overstimulated. For example, if a person has a traumatic brain injury, physical rehabilitation should be designed to rehab the brain as well. It is imperative to rehab the body appropriately for a person who may also have a traumatic brain injury. The body parts are associated with nerves that may recall trauma. If the patient also has post-traumatic stress disorder, it is imperative to treat the patient respecting the trauma.

A comprehensive body assessment is only the beginning of understanding the true depth of the dysfunctional body. Each rehabilitation session will provide more information to the practitioners so they can better diagnose and heal the patient. This is actually a great process because the more severe or complicated the injury, the more practitioners will learn about the dysfunction from multiple rehab sessions. It is also why healing takes time. Some injuries do not heal in the time pre-determined by insurance companies, doctors, or even some physical therapists.

I find this interesting as a scientist, because there are very few scientific laws that govern the universe. Everything else in this world is ever-changing. For example, Newton's first law states an object at rest remains at rest, while an object in motion continues its linear direction at constant velocity unless impacted by another object. This is why I view every injury as unique. There is no textbook injury. Setting a timeline or deadline on an injury will only lead to more dysfunction. For this reason, I recommend taking one's time and using tiny, incremental steps to provide the body time to heal naturally. It's pivotal to remember the body cannot be forced to heal faster than it is ready.

INCREMENTAL STEPS

POISE was designed to move at tiny, incremental steps. With a forward step, the team can analyze the functioning of the body. With backward steps, the team can eliminate inflammation and find the source of the injury. It also lets the therapist listen to the patient's body and experiment to find an alternate route to heal the patient. In addition, it allows for trauma to be part of the physical therapy process. It's key to move at a pace that balances both the physical healing and trauma release for the patient to heal.

In practice, the therapist should initially assign 1-5 reps (maximum reps) of an exercise. The therapist should never assign 15 reps initially. When the patient complains of pain or fatigue, the exercise should be ceased. The patient has reached their threshold.

The day after performing the maximum reps, the patient must evaluate their pain and soreness. If the patient feels no pain or soreness, the patient can repeat the exercise or wait another day before repeating the exercise. If the patient is able to quickly increase their repetitions, then they can proceed with caution. If the patient encounters pain, the patient is to follow pain protocol.

Pain protocol requires rest until the inflammation ceases. A variation of the exercise, such as dynamic stretches, with additional fascia manipulation may be assigned. Assign one rep of the exercise for day 1 and then allow the patient to evaluate their pain before continuing or increasing the repetitions over the following days. It may take months for the patient to build to five reps.

Therapy needs to be developed around the basics.

Mentally and physically, I felt a difference when I transitioned to doing weekly and biweekly 15-30 minute movement training sessions instead of twice weekly one-hour physical therapy sessions. In addition, my exercise therapist was able to focus on my application of the exercise in these sessions. We accomplished a lot in 15-30 minute sessions. My

THE MIRAGE OF POISE

exercise therapist had me fine-tune the exercises. Every little muscle was studied to verify that it was positioned correctly. It was painstaking work. I visualized each muscle for each exercise.

At the slower pace, I was able to question which muscle needed to be involved with each exercise. During a wall sit, for example, I could ask if I should feel my glutes or my inner thighs working. I was also able to focus on the position and engagement of the knees. With this new coaching philosophy, a whole 15 minutes would be spent with my exercise therapist on executing the wall sit.

As I executed the wall sit, I would continue explaining what I felt about the exercise to my exercise therapist. Most of the time, it was not what I should be feeling. Therefore, Active Edge would modify it and give me a new task or eliminate the exercise completely. If it appeared to be a forward direction, I would be assigned the exercise until my next appointment. Just because it was assigned and appeared to be forward progress did not mean it would continue to be forward progress once I began to do it on a more regular basis at home. In the end, POISE provided my exercise therapist the ability to listen to my body so we could work backward to find the root of my problems.

Static holds should rarely be used. Instead, dynamic stretches should be used. Sometimes static holds must be performed. In this case, I recommend starting with 3-5 second holds. When dealing with neurological and high-impact injuries, I recommend focusing on dynamic stretching.

A therapist should reconsider splitting exercises into variations to eventually put the whole exercise together. Variations of an exercise, such as plank variations or push-up variations, should be used to build to the larger, more comprehensive exercise. Another example was when Dr. Craner suggested working from the bottom up (Variation 1) and from the top down (Variation 2) to meet halfway to do a one-legged static lunge. For me, it took years of applying multiple variations, but eventually I was finally able to do some of the desired exercise. This technique led to me not only being able to be active, but also being able to begin running again.

PAIN WITH POISE

In addition, the patient should be advised to sit in proper posture. This definitely helps keep the back safer if there are concerns of a fractured spine and the spine surgeon chooses not to put the patient in a brace. This was highly challenging for me. I had so many weak back and core muscles; I was exhausted. It challenges the weak and atrophied regions of my legs that were injured in the accident. This is why I recommend proper posture as an actual rehabilitation exercise. Proper posture involves more than just the core muscles. It is a full-body exercise.

THE FOUNDATION OF POISE

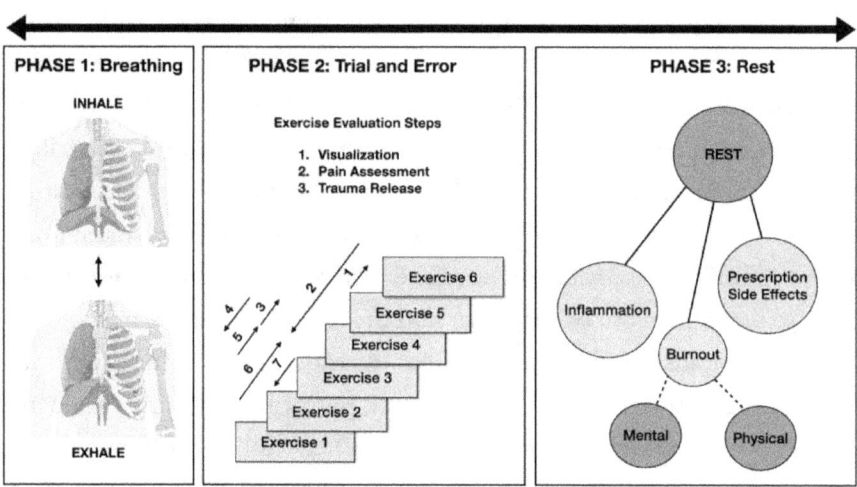

Figure 2. The success of rehabbing with POISE comes from building a foundation with PHASE 1 while achieving a balance between PHASE 2 and PHASE 3.[1]

The Foundation of Poise is shown in Figure 2. Phase 1 is the beginning of POISE rehabilitation. This is the breathing and visualization or mindfulness stage. It includes both establishing breathing dynamics and simultaneously benefiting from the mental aspects of mindful breathing.

Phase 2 is the physical rehabilitation stage. Each stair step represents an exercise of a certain skill level. During the exercise, visualization is used to help

THE MIRAGE OF POISE

determine issues. Trauma may also be released. Post-exercise, pain and trauma are evaluated. Then the physical therapist determines if the patient should move backward, remain at the current phase, or move forward in the rehabilitation plan. Each backward and forward arrow are used to indicate which direction the patient stepped in movement training in order to heal.

If it is necessary to take a step backward, then a backward arrow was used to indicate this movement. If the step was forward, then a forward arrow was used to indicate forward movement. However, even moving backward is still progress. Moving backward is just about more adequately placing the patient in the appropriate phase of injury to heal the patient. Basically, the patient had been at a too advanced stage of rehabilitation before that stage. This is why it's considered progression, even though it is "moving backward." This progress is shown in Figure 3, as each building block of a fine-tuned exercise develops each weakness into a functioning body.

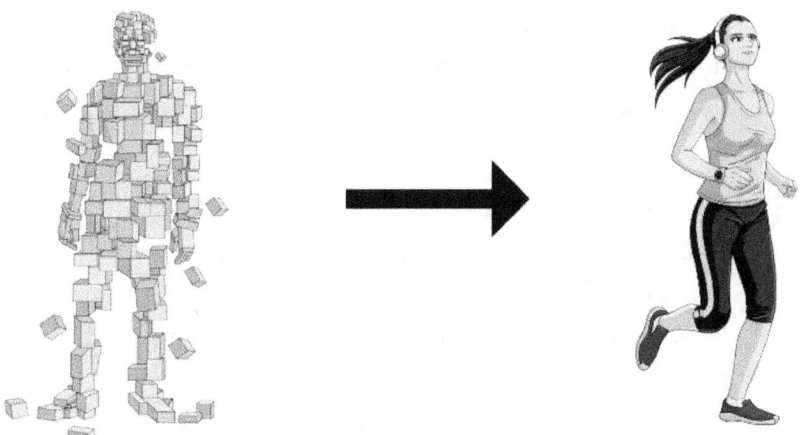

Figure 3. POISE recognizes healing the body is interconnected and is a complicated puzzle. A dysfunctional human is shown made of building blocks representing damaged body cells, tissues, fascia, etc. Some blocks have fallen (dysfunction) while others are not properly aligned (dysfunction). Applying all three phases of POISE will heal the whole body and eliminate dysfunction to achieve a functional human body. [2]

PAIN WITH POISE

Phase 3 is the rest period of POISE. Rest days are vital to any exercise routine. However, when in rehabilitation, a body needs even more rest. Rest should be considered necessary at the following times:

1. **If there is an inflammatory response resulting in pain after an exercise.** When an exercise triggers inflammation, especially of a nerve, the inflammation may cause burning, searing, pulling sensations, or even scream-worthy pain. This can require days of rest to allow the inflammation to dissipate. The exercise can be repeated with no modifications or with modifications, but with fewer repetitions. The goal is to do the exercise with no inflammatory response.

2. **When the patient is put on medications resulting in adverse side effects, such as fatigue, which could hinder therapy progress.** In cases like this, the patient must be given time to adjust. It can take a while to become adjusted to the medication. Therefore, adjusting physical therapy for this new fatigue should be considered for success of the physical rehabilitation program.

3. **The patient enters a phase of healing.** This could require additional rest due to the significant energy the body is using to rebuild after injury. This could happen when inflammation is suddenly removed from the body. However, the body needs time to repair it. It could also be the body needing to borrow energy from other body parts to focus on rebuilding the injured body part. The body only has so much energy to use. For this reason, the body may require rest.

4. **The patient endures burnout and must move at a slower pace for physical and mental health.** Burnout is interesting. Some people consider burnout as only psychological. However, a person's body can burnout as well. When a person does not

get the appropriate rest for their exercise regimen, the body can become inflamed and may even develop new injuries. This is why determining the person's injury status is vital to their rehabilitation plan.

To prevent burnout, totally revamp rehabilitation. Think of everything the sick patient is having to endure to heal. The sick person may be asked to sacrifice their life for multiple physical rehabilitation sessions, multiple doctor's appointments, at-home physical rehabilitation, and mental rehabilitation.

A patient is provided an uncertain time frame for injuries. Imaging only tells a partial picture of the injury. To heal the injury requires achieving a balance of easing and preventing inflammation, repairing damaged cells and fibers, and re-coordinating the mind-body. For me, I knew that traditional rehabilitation was overworking the body. For this reason, I think we are overdoing rehabilitation. Sometimes, less is more.

APPLICATION OF MINDFULNESS

Mindfulness was another vital component to my rehabilitation success. Incorporating mindfulness therapy should be at the foundation of any rehabilitation plan. It assists with visualization and breathing. It is great for stress reduction. I recommend applying mindfulness at the beginning of rehabilitation by using the breathing techniques. This will help build the breathing dynamic necessary for rehabilitation. Applying breathing exercises, like those used in mindfulness, will also help patients who have brain injuries, neurological dysfunction, and trauma by helping to breathe out the toxins and stress and breathe in fresh air using good posture.

The second part of mindfulness is visualization. Visualization should be used during physical therapy to assist in establishing the brain-muscle connection. It should also be used to envision doing an exercise correctly. This will help the body mimic the movement the brain pictures. It will also help find areas that may feel twisted, painful, tight, etc. Visualization can also be used in trauma therapy.

Visualization had its downsides, though. It could make a person realize the true reality of his situation. It could bring about extreme emotions. The day that someone is able to realize the true extent of damage sustained from an extreme injury is usually devastating. Most interestingly, for those who can achieve a true enlightenment, it requires an alternate perspective that awakens one's consciousness.

For example, my alternate perspective began when my brain finally fully comprehended what the body must do to overcome the injury. Part of this was the realization of what the body used to be able to do. The other part of this was realizing how much work was necessary to attempt to repair the damage to feel that way again. It was truly unthinkable what damage the tractor-trailer had done, and even more unthinkable what I was going to willingly put myself through to try and be active again. I was trying to accomplish the impossible. It was sadistic. It was maddening. It was all necessary to be an active, pain-free human again.

SUPPORT

During this time frame, friends and family are just as important as they are on day one. If a person needs distance from them, there are still ways they can provide support. If friends and family live a long distance away, it's pivotal for them to be creative and show support of some kind. Connection is vital beyond just a prayer. Send a card. Send flowers. Send a gif on the phone for a random surprise.

Sometimes the way to offer friends and family support during tough times is to provide food. Continue offering food after the person returns to work. As long as the person is recovering and still in rehab, providing food support is an option to consider.

THE MIRAGE OF POISE

Here are some ideas, especially if the family member or friend is long-distance.

1. Cook a meal and take it to the injured family member.
2. Buy gift cards for restaurants and send to the disabled friend.
3. Buy food at the grocery store for the exhausted family member and stock their refrigerator and freezer for them.
4. Cook homemade meals that can go in the freezer, and stock the disabled friend's freezer so there is food that can be pulled from the freezer.
5. Buy a meal from a restaurant and have it delivered.
6. Order food the disabled friend can put in the freezer and have it shipped to them. I learned there are amazing food options, such as lasagna, green beans, and mashed potatoes that can be ordered and shipped. They come in gluten-free options as well.
7. If the injured friend prefers healthy snacks, send a dried fruit and nut tray.

Finally, when a sick and disabled friend is anything but friendly, practice unconditional love. The sick friend needs rest and time to sort out what is going on in their sick body. A thick skin may be needed. A light-hearted attitude and smile are necessary. Anything heavy-burdened needs to be banned. When a person with trauma, high levels of pain, or a concussion needs to tune out, let them tune out. If a sick person reaches out, do as asked without delay. This will prevent the sick person from getting sicker.

Conversations that are uncomfortable for a sick person can weaken them. The toll of trying to process the topic can cause the person to pass out. The alternative to passing out is the sick person may scream, become combative, or leave the room and retreat. I don't say the latter to prevent these behaviors. I say this only to highlight this is how God made us.

PAIN WITH POISE

To become a more enlightened society requires we become more aware of how we communicate with the sick. We must learn how our words, tones, and actions affect the sick to prevent them from becoming sicker. The sick person is not a bully even in their most unruly stages. Instead, this behavior should be viewed as part of the injury. Pain is a bully, and the disabled person is trying to conquer the pain. I believe we, as a society, are far more exhausting to a sick person than we realize. We even unintentionally cause them harm by doing normal things like talking to them while ignoring how they may be feeling.

I argue not all things are meant to be fixed, including behavior. Attempting to fix all things will only exhaust the sick person and create an unwanted psychological complex.

I am very thankful my parents are stable and grounded. I am also very thankful I know myself. I'm not really sure where society developed the idea that an undesirable behavior needed immediate correction by another person. This delinquent discipline eliminates the ability of the human to learn how to self-discipline and self-correct. Society seems intolerant of others as they so eagerly enjoy correction of others. I learned society has become unable to laugh off mistakes. There is no learning curve for mistakes. There is no acceptance of mistakes. This was especially encountered in the medical field.

This was puzzling to me. At Chemical Abstracts Service, my annual assessment included professional objectives. One year, my manager assigned my professional objective to be "exhibit a learning curve for mistakes." This not only is necessary in a professional environment, but to develop as a leader, and even personally. This is the only way people can survive tough times.

A sick or injured person needs an environment that doesn't notice weaknesses or even mention them. The sick or injured person needs an environment where weaknesses may be necessary to be viewed as new strengths; an environment where mistakes can be laughed off and everyone

THE MIRAGE OF POISE

moves forward to another relaxing and enjoyable healing moment for the person. With the right mindset, being around a sick or injured person is not so scary, frustrating, or embarrassing.

BALANCE

Awareness and a new consideration of the intricate body, its energy, and its dysfunctions are necessary to heal this world. Applying SECCI (social, emotional, cultural, and contextual intelligences) when interacting with a sick or injured person will help anchor you, others around you, and the sick or injured person. It will provide a safe communication harbor for the sick person. It will provide a more stable environment for the sick person. It will help eliminate ego, pride, and bias. It will open the conscious to the sick person's needs without assuming what the need is. Assuming a person's need will only harm the sick person. These applications will also promote a safer, healthier environment so the sick or injured person can achieve balance.

As difficult as it may be, it's vital to accept that the sick or injured person is now different. After the accident, I was still fully functioning. This time, though, I had a disability. I had the same brain. It just needed to heal. I had the same body. It just needed to be put back together. I had the same soul. It just needed to evolve. However, I was treated differently than before the accident.

My dysfunctions resulted in people talking to me as if I was not as brilliant, that I should settle instead of challenging myself and taking risks, and it threw me into a new world of unconscious and conscious biases. For this reason, focusing on one's SECCI will greatly help the sick and injured person focus on his own SECCI by being in a low-stress environment, feeling empowered, and being his own voice in his rehabilitation.

Note: After trying lots of exercises, research, and discussion, the following are the exercises and rehabilitation plans that did the trick to let me reclaim my life. The next several chapters feature these exercises.

20.
BREATHING REHABILITATION

The tractor-trailer impacted my body and created almost a total core and shoulder instability, as well as spinal trauma. I suffered from trauma of my fascia, muscles, and nerves. My breathing functionality was traumatized as well. Therefore, when trying to function after the accident, I ran into unexpected issues with breathing at certain times. My breathing was more shallow, and attempts to breathe more deeply failed. Breathing would cause horrendous, sharp back pain, and I would feel my spine. The body's foundation rested upon functional breathing. As such, I had to rehab my breathing.

The first time I worked on my breathing was with my physical therapists at Location 2. I was told to breathe abdominally. I tried. I could not. When I tried to breathe abdominally, it felt like my lungs would not expand. I felt like I was suffocating. In fact, my chest felt like it was encased in concrete. My abdomen would not move. I felt like I was taking shallow breaths. When exhaling, I had better luck, but it was still a challenge.

Breathing during exercise was not foreign to me. In my exercise sessions prior to the accident, instructors would highlight breathing and sometimes would provide a new breathing technique. I also did yoga for years, which focused on breathing with the pose. I had even gone through running rehabilitation where I had been coached on breathing. I cycled through all the breathing techniques I knew and none of them worked.

After the accident, I received more suggestions from my physical therapists. One physical therapist wanted me to "suck in my stomach like I was at the beach in a swimsuit." It worked for my physical therapist just

PAIN WITH POISE

fine, and she was an excellent physical therapist. However, when I tried applying this breathing attempt, it didn't correct anything. This technique resulted in feeling like my spine was a rod. When trying to breathe with exercises, all of my back muscles, which were already an underlying source of pain, became even more inflamed. Attempting to breathe functionally with exercise was impossible to do.

There was something about my semi-trailer truck injury that was unique. Perhaps it was because it was an extreme impact injury, which resulted in an almost total instability of the core and shoulders. The injury involved a web of intricate fascia bands, which needed to be healed piece by piece. I was having to reconnect the muscles to the brain and retrain the muscles to work together. The techniques introduced in physical therapy were missing the puzzle pieces for this complicated injury.

To achieve functional breathing, I had to redevelop the breathing dynamic to move three-dimensionally[1] and involve the group of muscles in the core. This muscle group executed inhalation and exhalation. The muscles of the core include those of the rib cage, abdominal region, pelvic floor, spinal region, and the diaphragm. When healthy, the muscles of the rib cage, including the fascia, allow the rib cage to expand and contract. The rib cage moves anteriorly, laterally, and posteriorly.[2] When the muscle and fascia are healthy, the rib cage can freely expand. This allows maximum expansion of the lungs to fill with air. When injured, the muscles and fascia stiffen preventing the rib cage from expanding. This then prevents the lungs from fully expanding upon breath to fully fill with air.[3]

The muscles of the spine are attached to the rib cage. As the rib cage expands and contracts, the spine will extend and flex, respectively.[4] The remainder of the core moves like a balloon is being inflated or deflated with breath.[5] The diaphragm sits beneath the lungs. Upon inhalation, the lungs fill with air and push the diaphragm downward, as shown in Figure 4. The abdominal cavity and abdominal wall expand with inhalation. The pelvic floor lengthens and descends with the downward contraction of the diaphragm. With exhalation, the abdominal wall contracts to assist the abdominal cavity by forcing air out. This compresses the abdominal cavity. The diaphragm relaxes and moves upward, which forces air out of the lungs, as shown in Figure 4. At the same time, the pelvic floor will also contract and move upward.[6]

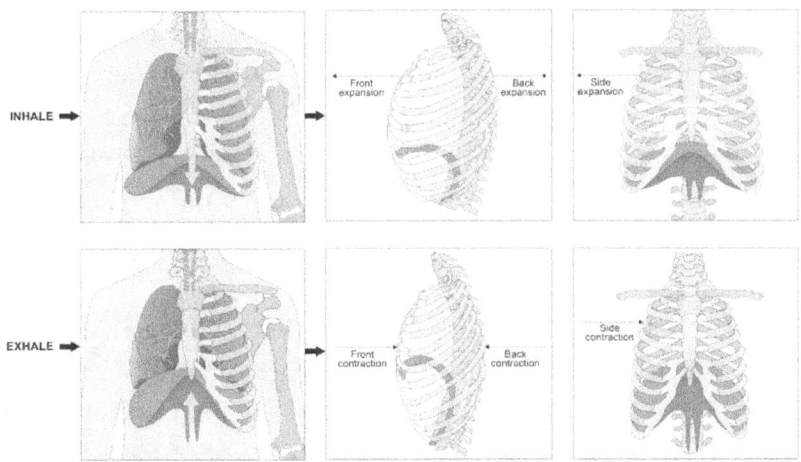

Figure 4. Upon inhale, the lungs fill with air so the diaphragm contracts downward. For three-dimensional breathing to occur upon inhale, the rib cage will expand in all three directions. Upon exhale, the lungs deflate upon exhale, so the diaphragm relaxes upward. For three-dimensional breathing to occur upon exhale, the rib cage will contract in all three directions.[7]

During my recovery, I was told by some physical therapists I was breathing incorrectly, because they noticed my chest moving while I breathed. I was told my abdomen was supposed to move with breath, but not my chest. This was perplexing to me. How could one's lungs fill with air if the chest wasn't allowed to move? When I changed my breathing after applying the following breathing techniques and began researching breathing functionality, I learned the chest was supposed to move. Then, my exercise therapist Olivia, CPT, SNC, SET, took it further and made me aware of breathing into my back. I never considered breathing into my back a thing until I had to do it to heal my dysfunction.

By fall of 2021, Olivia had introduced me to a new breathing technique. This breathing technique was adopted from James Fryer, NMT, LMT. I did this every day for months. It was literally the only exercise I did for months. Then, one day, I noticed a change. It had worked. My core felt like it was working together as one unit where all the pieces and parts were activating and functioning as one. When I began to try exercises I had put on hold for months, I was surprised at the ease with which I could perform them. I could also perform them with no pain or with little pain. Little did I know, I was reaching a new phase in my recovery that would really be eye opening. I was about to learn a lot.

When I began training for my first 5k in 2023, I began to learn even more about my breathing and movement dysfunction. While I needed to apply breathing techniques to begin my healing fundamentally, I also needed it to fine-tune my breathing with each advanced step of reclaiming my active life. In a perfect world, breathing techniques 1 and 2 (see instructions on following pages) may have resolved three-dimensional breathing alone. However, I found it impossible to breathe into my back on a hard surface while lying on my back. Standing and running were far more beneficial to retrain myself with three-dimensional breathing once I had initially rebuilt the core.

BREATHING REHABILITATION

BREATHING REHABILITATION EXERCISES

My healing relied on audible breathing. I call it "cah" breathing because that's what it sounds like when I make my sound. Therefore, I'll call it "cah" in this book.

Audible Breathing

Audible breathing is a type of diaphragmatic breathing. It is breathing that goes down the length of the trachea, engages the diaphragm, abdominal walls, and pelvic floor. I visualize air being scraped from the bottom of my abdomen just so I can best engage the abdominal and pelvic muscles. When the exhale begins, the audible noise, or "cah," begins. It should travel with the breath instead of staying in the throat. The breath motion will be slow. It should take at least 10 seconds from the initial audible breath to total release of all air and engagement of the pelvic floor for the audible breath to cease. Then "cah" is done.

Breathing Technique 1

Notes: I used breathing technique 1 to break up my rib cage. This assisted with loosening my fascia to allow my rib cage to lift and expand when I exhaled. It was a very painful movement when breaking up the fascia around the rib cage, but it was very useful. The exercise is also useful for retraining breathing if it is undesirable to break up the fascia around the rib cage.

Execution: Lie on the ground. If desired, place a small exercise ball between the knees. Lightly press the ball with the knees, but don't squeeze the ball. Inhale through the nose. Exhale through the mouth. On the exhale, perform audible breathing. It is of vital importance that the lower abdominal muscles be engaged even if it takes months to occur. Once all air is exhaled, hold for 2 seconds. Inhale through the nose. Relax. Then, jam the fingers under the rib cage. With the fingers curled under the rib cage on each side using both hands, move back and forth under both sides of the rib cage with the fingertips to break up the fascia.

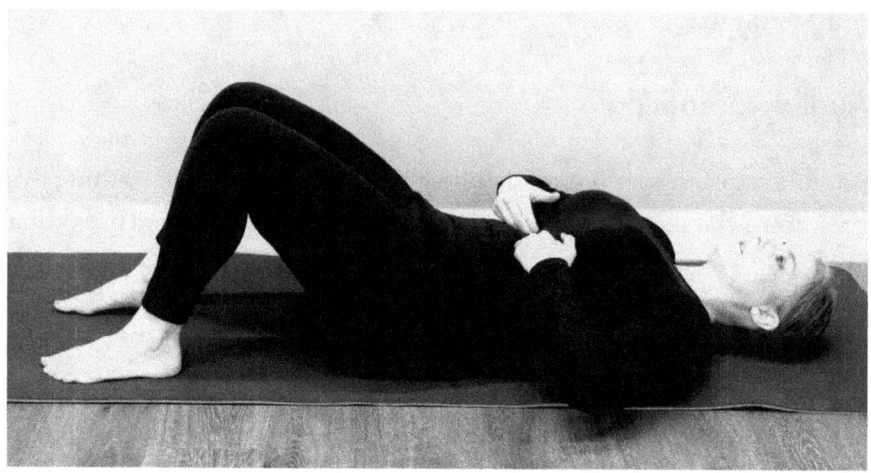

Figure 5. The model is shoving her fingers under her rib cage following breathing technique 1.

Once comfortable with breathing technique 1, move to Breathing Technique 2.

Breathing Technique 2

Notes: In 2019, my physical therapist wanted me to do a bridge pose variation for my lower body. Before the accident, I did bridge pose with my exercise routines. However, this time it wasn't working. My glutes were not functioning. My pelvis was not engaging with my core. And, I had no lower core involvement. Of course, I was supposed to breathe while performing the exercise and that wasn't happening either. In 2021, I was assigned this variation of bridge pose at Active Edge. It worked. Everything slid into place and reconnected. However, it took months.

BREATHING REHABILITATION

Execution: Variation 1. Lie on the ground. Place the heels on a step. Place a small exercise ball between the knees. Breathe in through the nose. Then, roll the pelvis slightly upward while exhaling using audible breathing.

Variation 2. Lie on the ground. Place the heels on a step. Place a small exercise ball between the knees. Breathe in through the nose. Then, roll the pelvis slightly upward, lifting the pelvis off the ground a little bit. While lifting the pelvis, exhale using audible breathing. Hold for 2 seconds. Lower.

Once comfortable with breathing technique 2, continue progressing.

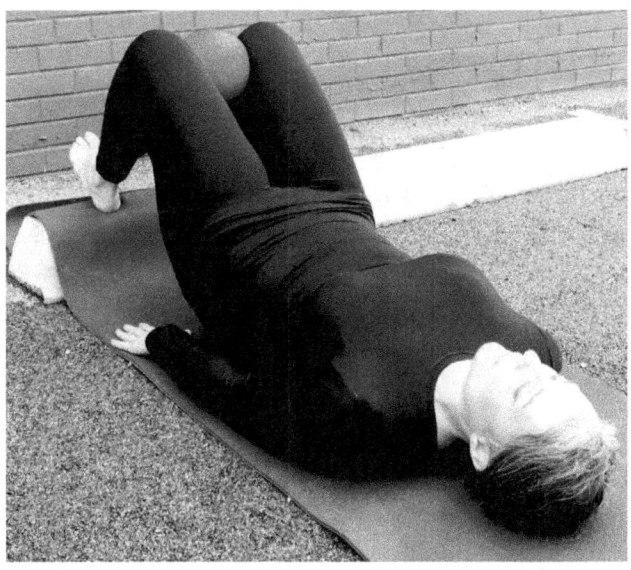

Figure 6. The model is lifting the pelvis upward in breathing technique 2.

Breathing Technique 3

Notes: After my first mile run resulted in unexpected spasms, Olivia suggested I was using a poor breathing pattern and was not using my upper thoracic for the inhale. She also didn't believe I was using my abdominals correctly for the exhale. Here is one exercise she suggested to correct my breathing dynamic.

Execution: Lie on the right side. Place a small exercise ball between the knees. On the inhale, breathe into the upper back so it moves slightly backward and expands. On the exhale, contract the obliques so the rib cage moves downward and inward. Repeat on the left side.

Then, replicate when running. Visualize the rib cage moving downward and inward on the exhale with the obliques tightening. Visualize the shoulder region expanding outward on the exhale.

Breathing Technique 4

Notes: After my first two-mile run, I told Olivia I could feel my rib cage struggling to shift with exhale breathing. She suggested this stretch prior to running to open the rib cage.

Execution: Lift the right arm. Then inhale into the rib cage. Visualize the rib cage expanding outward and enlarging with breath. Do not tilt to the left. Stay upright. Exhale. Switch sides. Repeat.

Breathing Technique 5

Notes: I ran my first two miles during training. My last mile was like running through quicksand. Plus, my eyes wanted to seep the whole time. Seep is the only word I have for it. It's not like a cry. I was beat up. I summarized my run and Olivia had more breathing exercises for me. This one really worked my weak legs, so I made sure to do a lot of repetitions. Yet again, there was nothing easy about this exercise.

BREATHING REHABILITATION

Execution: Take the exercise ball and place it against a wall. Kneel on the hands and knees. Place the feet so they are angled toward each other and under the edge of the exercise ball. The ball should not rest on the feet or legs. Move the buttocks toward the ball so the buttocks lightly touch the exercise ball. The buttocks should not press into the exercise ball. Inhale. Using the inhale, move away from the ball. Then, exhale toward the ball. Touch the buttocks to the ball. Use the core to move instead of using the legs.

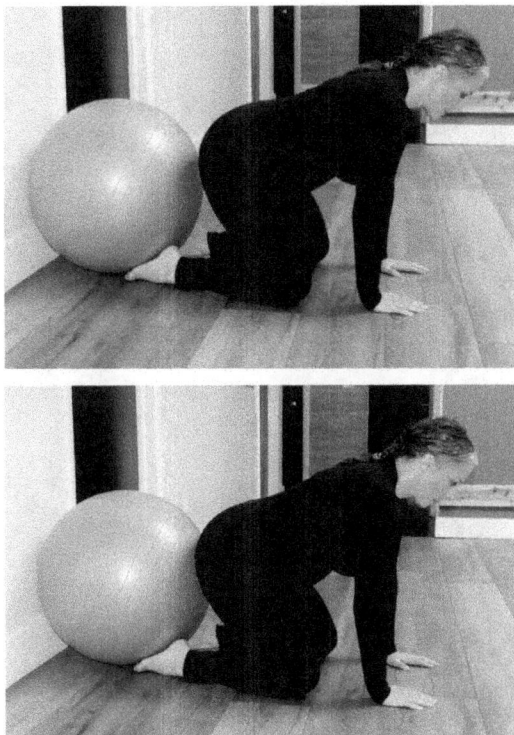

Figure 7. (*Top to bottom*) The model is in starting position of breathing technique 5; the model is moving toward the exercise ball.

21.
CORE REHABILITATION

At first, my rehabilitation after the accident was all about the neck. What we did not learn at Location 2 was that I could not rotate my back without increasing my pain levels. Location 2 failed to realize I had no core strength. Each twist of my back resulted in pain so severe I could feel the pain in the middle of my back along my spine. I would often say during this time I could feel my spinal cord. I was told this was not the truth, but that's what it felt like. Eventually, my exercises revolved around what was safe for my back as well. This began a new phase of healing and enlightenment about my injuries.

When Dr. Josh Murphy diagnosed me with "almost total core instability," I knew I had found a doctor who understood my injuries. Dr. Murphy explained core instability as a core that was not functioning normally due to an unknown cause. Kathi Bushway, COTA/L at Essentrics® describes the core as the region of the body that is confined at the top by the diaphragm, the bottom by the pelvic floor, the front and sides by the deep abdominal muscles, and the back by the deep spinal muscles.[1]

When a body part does not function normally, another body part responds to assist it. Sometimes, pain may result. Causes of dysfunction may be a muscle sprain, muscle tear, ligament damage, etc. I had spent six months in physical therapy with no results. Since all the traditional core exercises assigned were not getting to the root of the issue, Dr. Murphy began the process of determining the root of my dysfunction.

PAIN WITH POISE

Dr. Murphy immediately had me stop doing all the exercises I had been assigned in physical therapy. I was to rest as I was inflamed from just doing my physical therapy exercises. Over the next year, Dr. Murphy began evaluating exercises to rebuild my core, provided guidance with my physical therapy, and monitored my at-home rehabilitation. The process of repair proved to be very difficult. I was facing the challenge of rebuilding my core with an injured neck and shoulders. I was assigned inclined push-ups against the wall. He provided tips to assist or correct what my physical therapist was assigning.

Upon transitioning to Active Edge, I continued in the fall of 2020 with a much stricter rehabilitation of my core. We began with my squat form as I wanted to do squats. Dr. Craner evaluated my squat form. I knew I wasn't doing them correctly. My groin was still screaming. She tried some modifications. I added these modifications to my regular rehabilitation routine from my pre-COVID therapists. Then, I met Olivia.

Over the next few months, my team added one exercise at a time to my rehabilitation plan. Olivia would eliminate the exercises that were determined to be above my wellness status, which was essentially everything assigned during rehabilitation. After careful evaluation, the Active Edge team discovered my body parts were still not wanting to work together. With lots of experimentation, the rehabilitation plan became applying breathing techniques with movement training at a 10-degree pace.

In order to rehabilitate the core, I had to integrate spine rehabilitation with breathing rehabilitation, and leg and foot rehabilitation. I also needed to rehab my neck. The back muscles are connected to the neck muscles, to the abdominals, and to the pelvic floor. Because the muscles and fascia of the neck are connected to the muscles and fascia of the back, we had to consider the whole body to heal my neck. I don't know if we can say what happened first—whether the neck injury caused injuries throughout my body as my body tried to save my neck. I don't know if we

CORE REHABILITATION

can say the core was destroyed first by trying to save my neck and other body parts. What I did know was the core needed to be rehabbed, and by focusing on rehabbing my core, it made it easier to rehab everything else. However, it required the right kind of rehab.

CORE REHABILITATION EXERCISES

Clamshells

Notes: I was assigned this exercise at Location 3. I didn't progress quickly. However, I did improve over the years. I didn't find that the breathing techniques necessarily improved this exercise.

Execution: Lie on one side with the knees bent. Keeping the legs bent at the knees, raise them into the air. Open the legs while keeping the feet together. Close the legs to return to the starting position. The legs should not completely close. Be careful to not engage the neck.

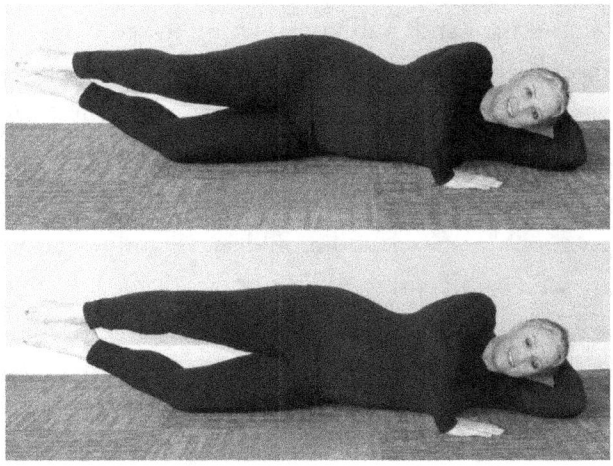

Figure 8. (*Top to bottom*) The model is preparing to perform a clamshell; the model is performing a fully opened clamshell.

PAIN WITH POISE

Cow pose

Notes: This was one of the first exercises assigned during rehabilitation. While I used to love this pose before the accident and practiced it daily, it caused pain and discomfort after the accident. Each chiropractor wanted me to perform cow pose as well. However, I stopped doing it because it was so painful. I hope this drastic change of before and after the accident highlights the unique pain experienced in this injury. It was indescribable.

As a teenager, I had low back pain. I fixed that with exercise, and it permanently went away. That pain was a 1 compared to this pain level being a 10 for years. Even when I had an inverted lumbar, I could go hiking. The pain for the inverted lumbar was a 1. Tractor-trailer back pain was off the charts pain. Once I rebuilt my foundation using breathing techniques 1-2, I was able to perform cow pose again. I may have still had limited flexibility, but I was finally able to perform the exercise pain-free.

Hint: The key to this exercise is to only use the core to curl.

Execution: Get on the hands and knees. Using the core only, roll the core upward so the back curls toward the ceiling. Be careful to not roll upward using the back or shoulders, as these will naturally roll as the abdomen rotates upward. Then, roll the abdomen down toward the floor. When rolling the abdomen, engage the lower abdomen on the upward and downward rotations. The back and shoulders will only slightly curl, unlike the abdomen, which will curl significantly.

CORE REHABILITATION

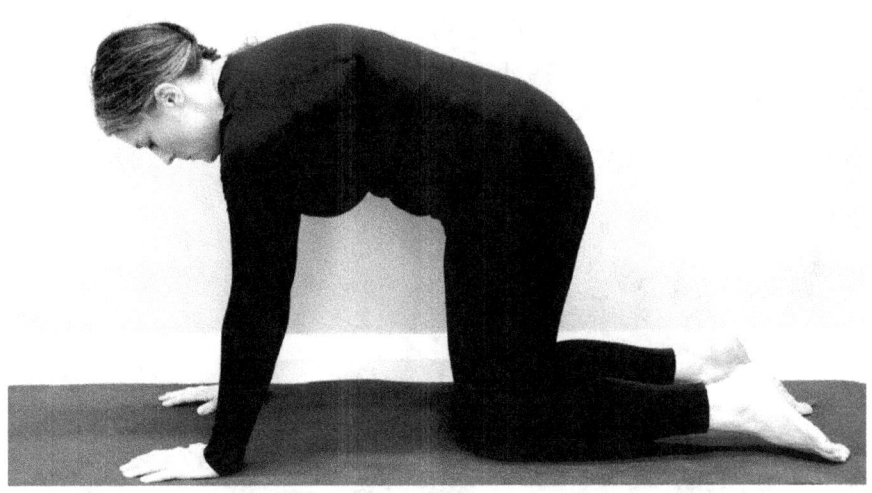

Figure 9. The model is curling upward in cow pose.

Elbow planks

Notes: I began doing elbow planks in 2019. However, I knew I was in a lot of pain. Eventually, I determined the elbow planks were worsening my facial spasms and temporomandibular joint (TMJ) issues. I tried to reduce full elbow planks to elbow planks on my knees, but I still encountered the same issue. My chiropractor had me correct my upper body form with a simple modification. This correction in my form was pivotal to rebuilding my upper back, neck, and core muscles.

Execution: Dr. Craner's modification: Stand upright with arms in an L-shape by sides. Visualize the arms being pulled downward but without actually moving them. This creates a flat back. To mimic the upright position, visualize the arm muscles in the lower arm pulling backward or "sliding" but without actually dragging the lower arms along the floor. This action straightens the back.

Variation 1: Lie on the floor. Then, get on the elbows and knees just like in a push-up position with the body fully extended. Apply Dr. Craner's modification to the arms. Be sure to not engage the neck or face muscles, which will tighten the muscles. Build up to a 30-second hold.

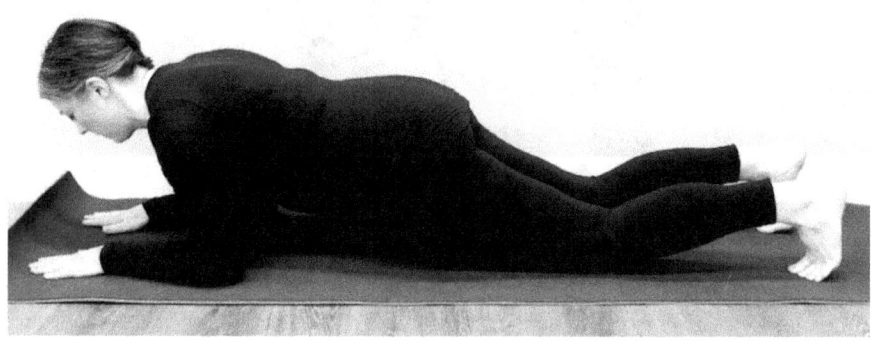

Figure 10. The model performs elbow plank with the knees on the floor.

Variation 2: As the core strength and back muscles improve in strength, move to full elbow plank by lifting the knees off the floor.

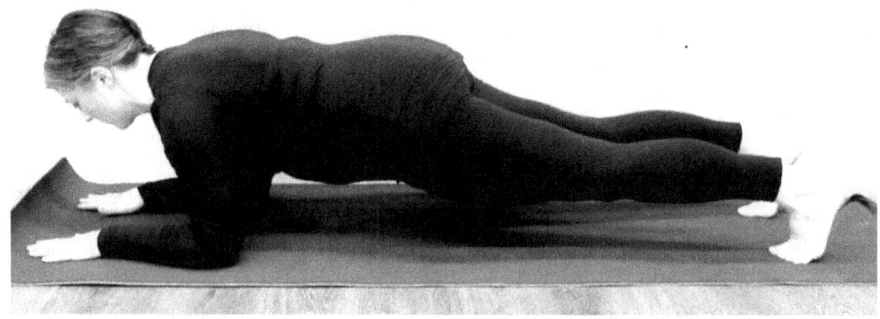

Figure 11. Elbow plank is shown in full extension.

CORE REHABILITATION

Reverse Clamshells

Notes: I was assigned this exercise in 2019 at Location 3. For the reverse clamshell, a pillow can be inserted between the knees.

Execution: Lie on one side with the knees bent. Bend the top leg at the knees to raise the lower leg into the air. Be careful to not engage the neck. Lower the top leg.

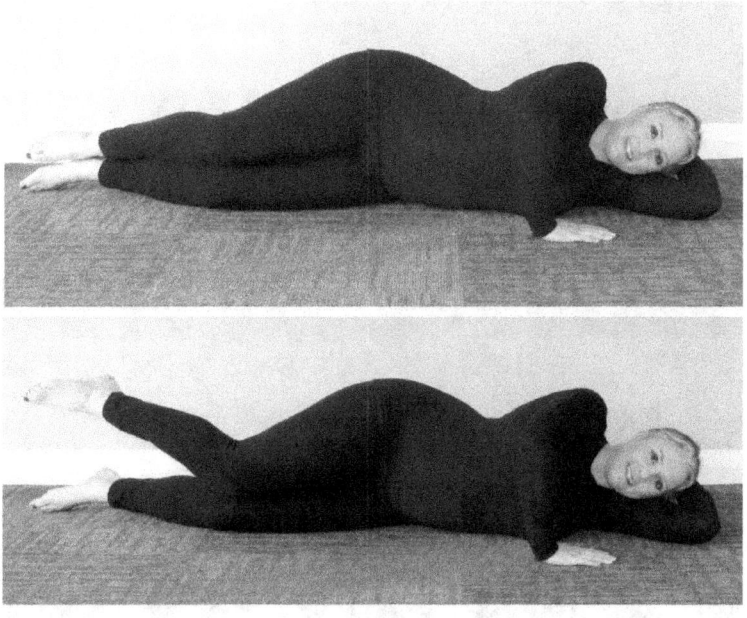

Figure 12. (*Top to Bottom*) The model is preparing to perform a reverse clamshell; the model is performing a fully opened reverse clamshell.

Side Leg Lift

Notes: When I began this exercise, I could barely lift my top leg. I was assigned this exercise at Location 3 in 2019. As of 2023, I could do 30 reps before fatiguing.

Execution: Lie on one side. Raise the top leg. To extend the leg during the lift, extend the toes away from the head. Be careful to not engage the neck. Extend out of the hip joint. Lower the leg.

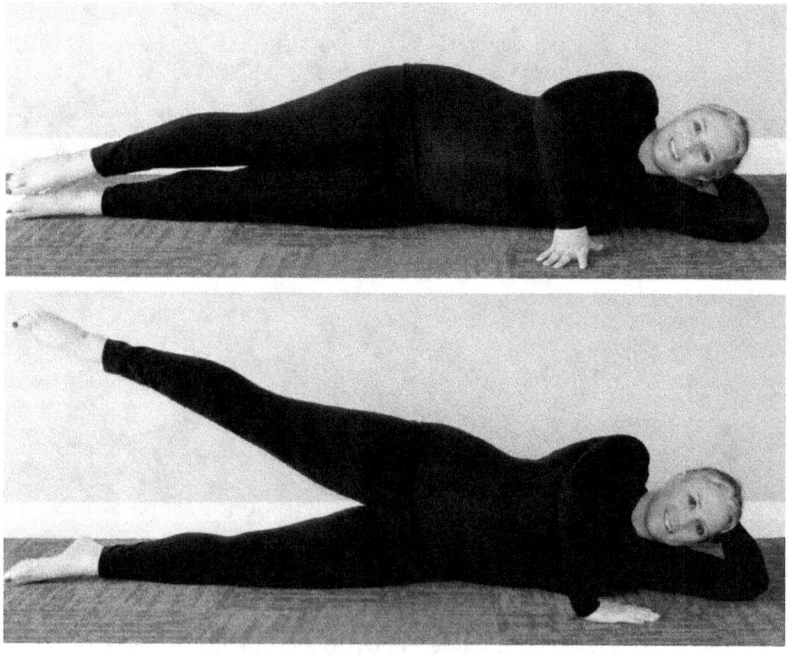

Figure 13. (Top to bottom) The model is in starting pose; the model is executing side leg lift.

CORE REHABILITATION

Skin Sliding

Notes: Practicing skin sliding was uncomfortable, but it was useful as it massaged the muscles and fascia. The stomach is a great area to skin slide. I also highly recommend practicing skin sliding on the chest.

Tip: Go deep. Even though it's called skin sliding, it actually gathers the skin and fat layers.

Execution: Gather a large amount of skin in the fingers and knead it like dough. Then, move to another area to skin slide.

Bicycles

Notes: I began the modified bicycle in fall 2023. I came up with this variation on my own. It helped build my core and improve my breathing.

Execution: Lie facing up on the floor with the upper body elevated on the forearms. Raise the legs into a bent position. Engage the core and breathe into the thoracic cavity. Be sure the upper back moves with breathing. Cycle the legs. With the exhale, be careful to not engage the neck. Use the lower core muscles.

Spine Twist

Notes: This is a great exercise to begin building rotation of the upper body. I always rotated from the abdomen, even in yoga prior to the accident. I thought this was safe. Then, after the accident, this hurt my back and spine. I still wanted to rotate my upper body, though. I loved spinal twists, especially in yoga. I asked Dr. Craner what I should do. This is the tip Dr. Craner suggested. It was pain-free for me.

Execution: Stand straight. Then, visualize the spine. Rotate the upper body by rotating from the spine. The neck must stay in alignment with the spine.

PAIN WITH POISE

Foam Roller

Notes: I could not foam roll after the accident. Dr. Craner suggested this alternative.

Execution: Start with the foam roller at shoulder height. Lie on the floor with the foam roller under the shoulders. The foam roller should be under the full width of the upper back. Bend the knees. Place the hands clasped behind the head. Dip the buttocks to the ground and rest it on the ground. Lower the head, neck, and shoulders toward the ground. Keep the rib cage together. Hold. Then, lift the head and buttocks. Roll the foam roller down a few inches. Repeat the dip of the buttocks and lowering of the head. Hold. Repeat for the length of the spine.

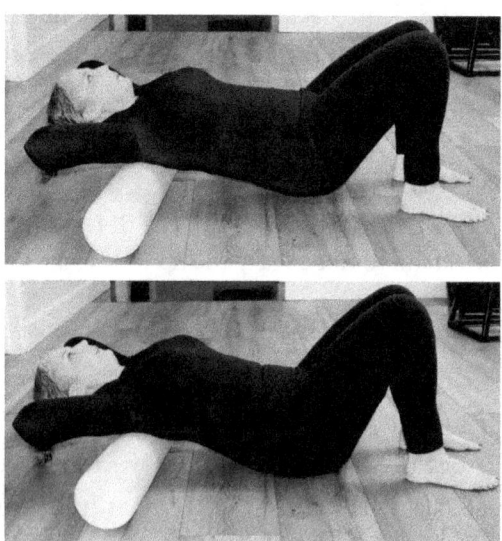

Figure 14. (*Top to bottom*) The model is in the upright position of the foam roller variation; The model is in the lower position.

CORE REHABILITATION

Bird Dogs

Notes: Alternating lifting arms and legs during a plank was very popular in my rehabilitation plan. However, it failed. It didn't matter who assigned it, such as chiropractors or physical therapists, the number of attempts, or the therapies I attended. Even with Dr. Murphy telling me to take breaks from them and then starting me up with the exercise again after additional rehabilitation, it still didn't work. The exercise was causing me pain and it was not as I remembered pre-accident. Quite frankly, that's all my brain could really do. It sent alerts to me saying, "Something is wrong." Then, Olivia tried something new in 2021. She introduced me to bird dogs. These were very challenging, but I could do them.

Execution: Kneel on the hands and knees. Then, tuck the pelvis under slightly. This is the key to the exercise. While keeping the pelvis tucked, raise the left arm off the ground and the right leg off the ground. Keep the right leg bent. The right leg will likely not extend far. This is okay. The left arm may not be straight or move off the ground far. This is okay. Return to the ground. Then, do the opposite side. Be careful to not lean to one side when lifting the arm and leg off the ground. Keep the pelvis and back level.

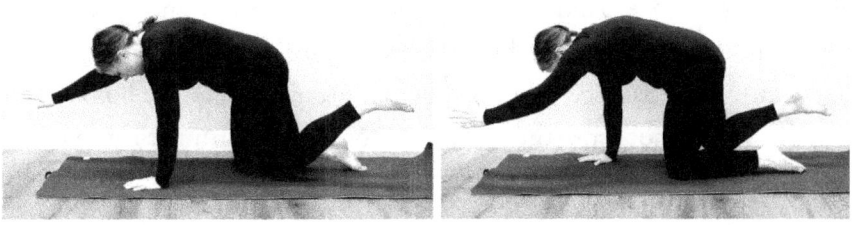

Figure 15. (Left to right) The model performs bird dog alternating right arm and left leg; the model performs bird dog alternating left arm and right leg.

Hamstring Stretch

Notes: This exercise was a stretch I did as a runner. It was an easy stretch until I was hit by an 18-wheeler. As it required upper body strength, it was an exhausting stretch. Four years later after lots of healing, it's a great stretch and easy for me to do again. Therapists should consider upper body strength before assigning it.

Execution: Lie with the legs extended along the floor. Place the right foot in a resistance band. Extend the right leg toward the ceiling holding tension in the resistance band with the right hand. Keep it as straight as possible. Then, pull the right leg toward the floor. Quickly pull it back up using the hip joint. Do 10-15 quick repetitions to loosen the muscles. Then, slightly pull the foot and leg toward the head using the resistance band, if able. Hold.

Place the left hand on the left hip to anchor the left hip. The hip should not move. Then, shift the right leg toward the outer right side. Hold with the resistance band. Evenly use the abdominals to hold the leg. Breathe and do not tense the neck, jaws, or face. If necessary, rest the leg on a chair for support.

Shift the resistance band to the left hand. Place the right hand on the right hip. Anchor the right hip. Shift the right leg toward the left side. Hold with the resistance band. Evenly use the abdominals to hold the leg. Breathe and do not tense the neck, jaws, or face. Return the leg to extend toward the ceiling before releasing to the floor.

Repeat with the left leg.

CORE REHABILITATION

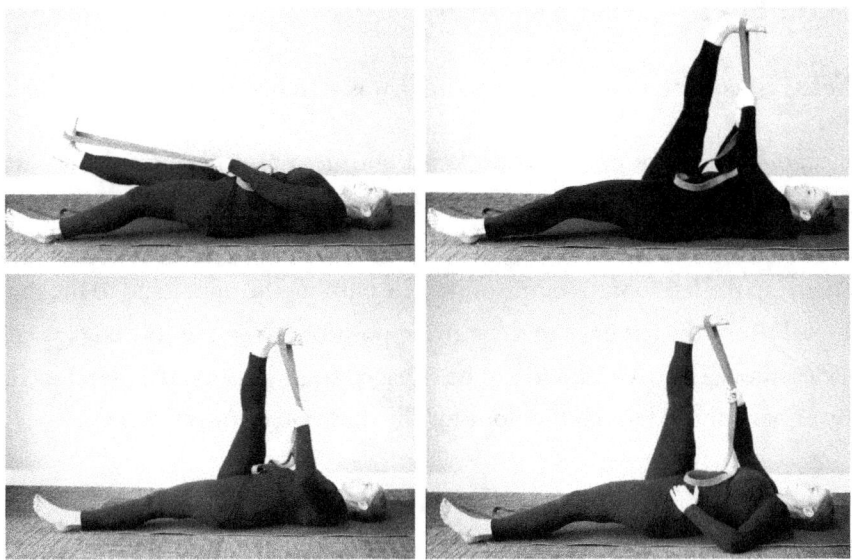

Figure 16. The model shows various stages of hamstring stretch. *(Clockwise from left)* The right leg is stretched down; the right leg is stretched to the ceiling; the right leg is stretched right; the right leg is stretched left across the body.

Jumping Jack

Notes: In 2021, I was finally able to add the jumping jack to my routine. To say I was excited was an understatement. I had to build my core and legs to handle the exercise. Before, landing when jumping resulted in feeling every vertebra in my spine. It felt like brick upon brick. I considered jumping jacks to be one step closer to running again.

Execution: Stand with the feet a few inches apart with arms to the side. Jump the feet hip width apart while moving the arms upward in a V-position. Jump the feet back to the starting position with arms returning to the sides.

Dead Bugs

Notes: To continue building my core, I was assigned dead bugs by Olivia.

Execution: Lie back on the floor. Bend both legs together into the air as if sitting in a chair. Then, tap the right foot to the ground while tapping the left hand to the left knee. Raise the right knee back to the starting position. Then, tap the left foot to the ground while tapping the right hand to the right knee. Return the left knee to the starting position. Keep the core engaged for the exercise. The neck should not be engaged (tight) during the exercise. The lower back should touch the floor for the duration of the exercise.

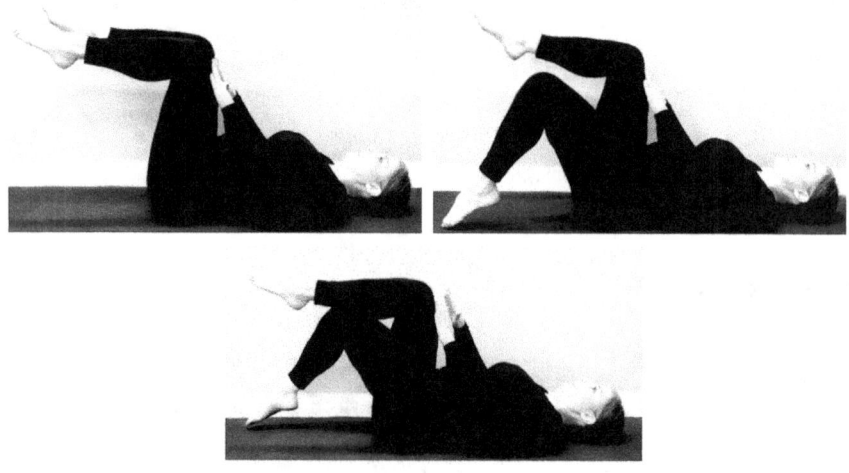

Figure 17. The model performs various stages of dead bug. *(Clockwise from left)* The model is in start position; the model is tapping right hand to right knee; the model is tapping left hand to left knee.

CORE REHABILITATION

Leg Lifts

Notes: When I started doing leg lifts in Pilates, I realized I couldn't get my body parts to connect and engage even with the assistance from the Reformer Apparatus.® I mentioned it to Olivia. My major complaint was the disconnect in the abdominal region. My left side was not engaging. Every once in a while, with a lot of thinking and visioning of the abdominal region, it felt like it would pull together and work. However, the effort was extreme. I could also tell the difference between the left side and the right side. We tried a few things. Once I rebuilt my foundation using breathing techniques 1-2, this exercise became as easy to perform as before the semi-trailer truck.

Execution: Lie with the back against the floor. Then, lift the right leg toward the ceiling. Keep the abdominals and pelvic floor engaged with the back stabilized against the floor. Lower the right leg. Then, repeat the exercise with the left leg.

BUILDING TO A CRUNCH

I had a back injury, and one physical therapist thought I would never run again. She even told me she didn't think I would be able to do kettlebells. Well, I wasn't going to listen to anything negative. I had dreams. I was going to break those walls. This meant I had to curl my back again. I had to rotate it. I also had to be able to take jolts every time I landed. I needed to be able to bounce again without feeling it in my back like bricks. Of course, this meant rebuilding my core but also healing damaged fascia, muscles, and increasing my flexibility. In 2021, I started to build up to performing a crunch.

Elbow to Knee

Notes: I found this exercise particularly helpful as it stretched and aided in flexibility of my core. My core was inflexible and it was difficult to move from side to side. I basically moved like a stiff rod. This exercise helped my back and neck more than cow pose.

Execution: Kneel on the knees. Get in position for child pose. Then, place the opposite elbow against a knee. Keep the hips level.

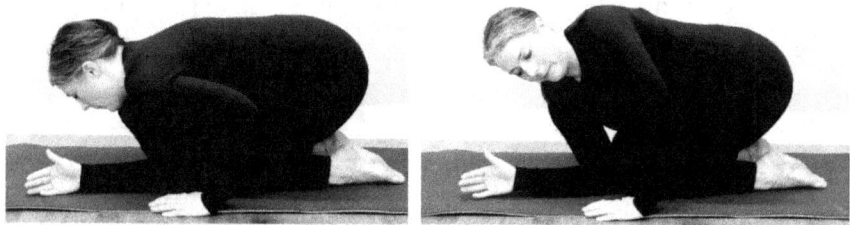

Figure 18. (*Left to right*) The starting pose of elbow to knee is shown. The model touches elbow to knee.

CORE REHABILITATION

Standing Elbow to Opposite Hip Crunch

Notes: I was not able to do elbow to opposite hip crunches on my back. However, I could do them standing. Once I rebuilt my foundation using breathing techniques 1-2, this became a very simple exercise unless I had a spasm.

Execution: While standing, place the right hand behind the neck. Without pulling on the neck, roll downward toward the opposite hip with the core. Get as close to the opposite hip with the elbow as possible. Hold at final position and exhale completely. Return to the starting position. Switch sides. Repeat.

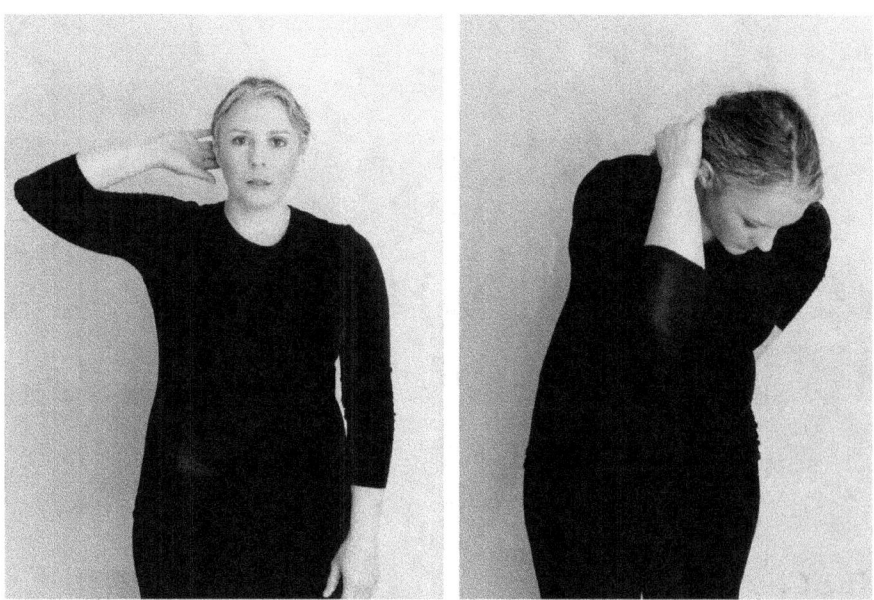

Figure 19. (*Left to Right*) The model is in starting position of standing elbow to opposite hip crunch; the model moves her left elbow to her right hip.

Engage the Core

Notes: This is a preparation step for the crunch pose.

Execution: Lie with the back flat against the ground. Put a small exercise ball between the knees. Then, engage the core muscles to prepare for the crunch without lifting. Think of the abdominal wall, obliques, lower abdominals and pelvic floor when engaging the core. Do not tighten the neck or back. Release. Do this several times. Continue to do this exercise while building up to slowly lifting the head and shoulders off the ground, if possible.

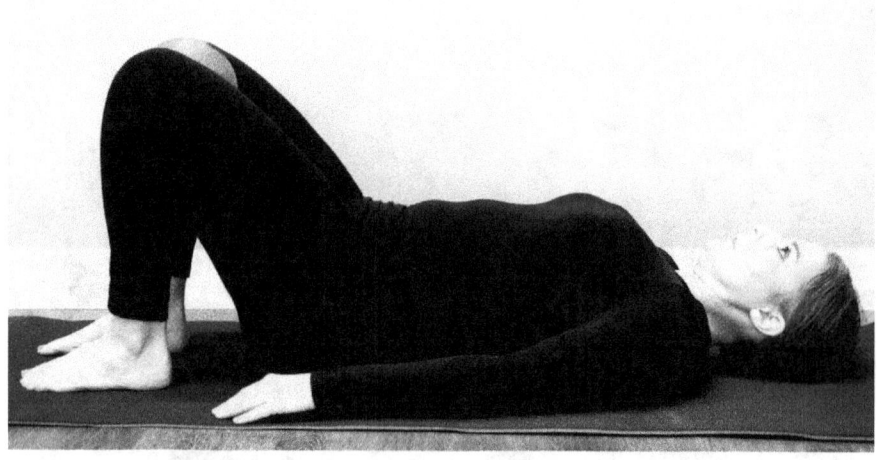

Figure 20. The model is engaging her core using an exercise ball between her knees.

The Crunch

Notes: By 2022, I was finally able to attempt the crunch. I learned that an injured body part was more susceptible to environmental factors and personal factors. Therefore, functioning of the human body varied even more on a daily basis when injured. Some days I couldn't do a crunch. Other

CORE REHABILITATION

days, I felt great doing a crunch. As of 2023, I felt great doing crunches and could do 20 crunches at a time. However, that was overdoing it for my body, because I would suffer from spasms and nerve pain for days. The pain was horrendous. I would have to find a balance.

Execution: Lie on the ground. Bend the legs. Put an exercise ball between the knees. Then, engage the core to prepare for the crunch lift. First, lift with the upper chest. Focus on lifting from the breastbone. This will relax the neck when lifting from this region of the upper chest. Then, continue the crunch curl by engaging the lower abdomen. Exhale. Lower the upper body with the abdominal muscles. Inhale on the way down. Repeat.

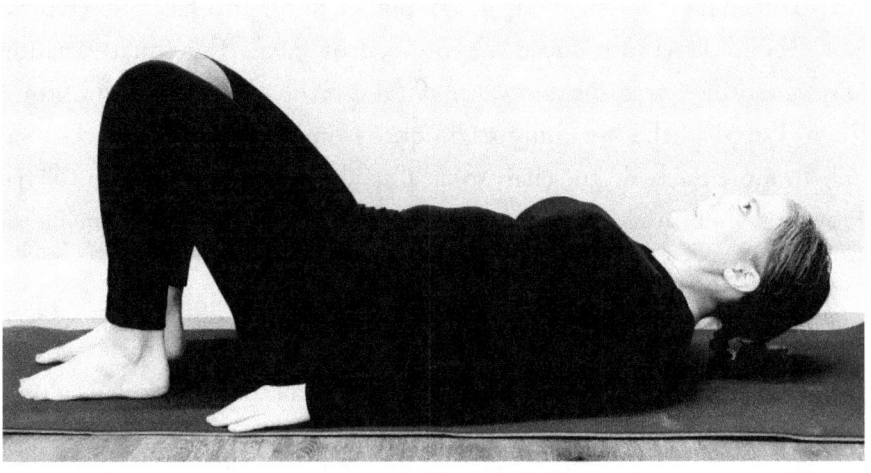

Figure 21. The crunch.

BUILDING TO A SINGLE LEG STATIC LUNGE

When I was at physical therapy location 2, I had only been diagnosed with a neck injury, even though I had persistent pain in my groin. I asked my physical therapist if I could do squats. At the time, she didn't know why

PAIN WITH POISE

I couldn't. I had been doing squats prior to the accident and had to squat regularly at my job at Kohl's. Squatting was something I was quite efficient at doing. I thought it would resolve my groin pain. Unfortunately, this idea failed. I stopped immediately with squats in 2018.

Through the years, I attempted to get a diagnosis. It failed. I attempted to get physical therapy for the region. I was told I would never run again. Then, when I went to Active Edge in 2020, Dr. Craner re-evaluated my squats. Dr. Craner wanted me to practice doing a squat facing the wall. By doing this isolated version, we realized I could not perform a squat. I was told to put books on a stair step and practice sitting down on it with my knees at the same angle as my ankles and to squeeze my glutes together to rise. That didn't work. Another method involved squatting a few inches away from a wall. The goal was to maintain my upper body in appropriate form. That failed miserably.

Then, Olivia introduced me to the chair squat. This squat variation was something I was able to do even if it did involve a lot of modifications. Then, I applied the breathing techniques from James Fryer. Soon, I was able to more easily do the chair squat I had been working on with Olivia. However, I still wasn't doing it right. The chair squat only got me closer to proper squat form.

In the meantime, I wanted to do a single leg static lunge. I used to do these regularly in my leg workout. Dr. Craner started me on the 10-degree approach of building to a single leg static lunge. I still could not feel my glutes, especially the very bottom of my glutes, when I began working on the single leg static lunge in 2020. There was a distinct disconnect from my glutes to my hamstrings, and it was just numb. This numbness wasn't just nerve. It was atrophied muscle. I had a long road.

Dr. Craner developed a plan. The goal was to meet in the middle. I was to start at the bottom and build the muscles with the leg lunge pushup. I was to start in a lower position from a normal leg lunge position. The goal was to eventually meet in the middle. As of 2023, I am still building on meeting in the middle.

CORE REHABILITATION

Wall Sit

Notes: Use a small exercise ball for this exercise.

Execution: Stand with the feet a few inches away from a wall. Place the small exercise ball between the knees. Plant the large toes on the floor. Don't grip with the toes, though. Maintain the core so the lower body and the neck are both flat against the wall. On the exhale, slide down the wall. Lower until in a chair position, if possible. Use the inner thighs instead of the buttocks for the position. Hold. Return to standing. Repeat.

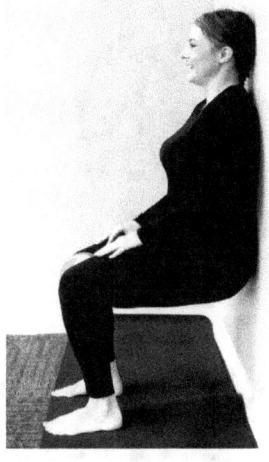

Figure 22. The wall sit.

Deadlift

Notes: I did deadlifts before the accident. In 2021, I inquired about deadlifts. My hamstrings and lower back muscles were extremely weak. I thought deadlifts might be the answer to target them. Active Edge showed me two variations.

PAIN WITH POISE

Execution:

Variation 1: Stand with the feet hip distance apart. Hold a straight object, like a pole or broom, along the spine to keep the back straight. Bend the knees slightly. Hinge forward at the hips keeping the core engaged. Let the upper body lower toward the floor without curling the back. Then, lift from the core and hips to return to the starting position.

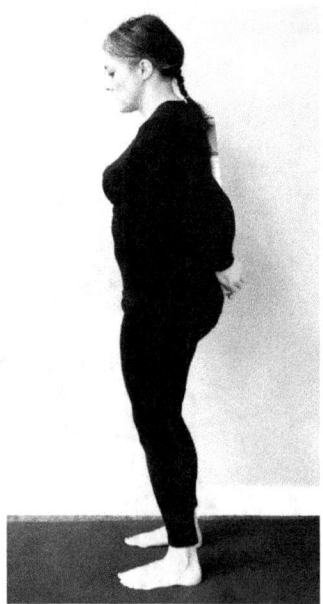

Figure 23. The model is showing variation 1 of the deadlift. A straight object is aligned along the spine.

Variation 2: Stand with feet hip distance apart. Bend slightly at the knees. Hinge forward at the hips and not with the back. Lower the upper body toward the floor, keeping the back straight and the shoulder region relaxed. Do not tighten the back muscles. Keep the core engaged. The shoulders will curl forward slightly, but the back will not curl. Then, return to the starting position using the core, hamstrings, and glutes. The back should stay relaxed.

CORE REHABILITATION

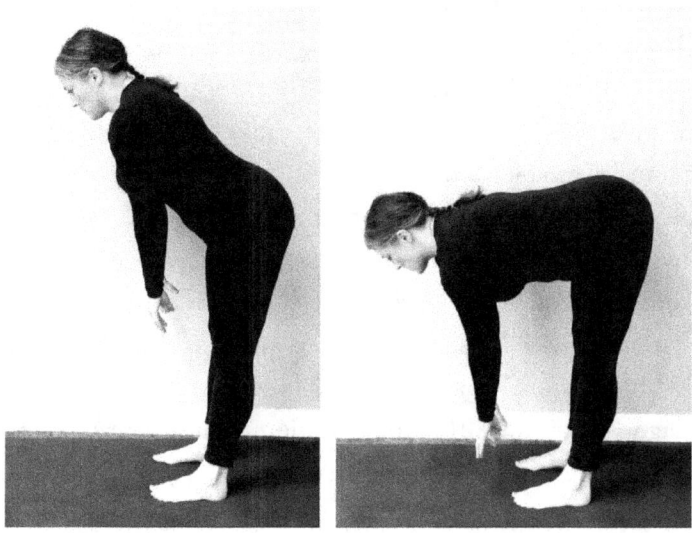

Figure 24. The model is performing stages of variation 2 of the deadlift.

Single Leg Push-up

Notes: I was first assigned this exercise in May of 2021. When I did this exercise, I learned the difference between my two legs. When my right knee was on the ground, the most worked and most weak muscles were those of my inner thigh along my groin injury. When my left knee was on the floor, the worst of the exercised muscles were on the outer edge and the region just above my knee where the bruise had been, which was indicating the weakest muscles. In addition, I had to squeeze my glutes together with much more effort to even raise myself off the floor and was doing so with almost all of my upper body weight supported on a raised object. My left leg fatigued after 2 attempts, and I limped around the house needing assistance walking.

As I challenged myself more and more with increasing repetitions and using more of my own body weight, I eventually hit a trauma wall.

PAIN WITH POISE

I kept hitting the trauma wall until I screamed one night working my left leg. It was a special scream. I had triggered trauma. Then, I processed trauma immediately after the exercise. This repeated for a bit but not to the same extreme. After a few months, something finally clicked back together and I was able to do the exercise more regularly and with more ease. I also experienced trauma less often.

However, the pain in the left side of my head became too severe for me to do any single leg push-ups. The left side of my head endured the most trauma as it was impacted by items during the crash. I have nerve irritability and damage, possible blood vessel damage, migraines, and undiagnosed trauma. This complication means there are days, even in 2023, when doing one leg lift is debilitating.

Execution: Kneel on the ground beside a support. The best support will allow placement of both hands for even weight support, such as a chair on either side of the body. Place one hand on each chair. Lift the right leg and keep it bent at a 90-degree angle so the foot is planted on the floor. Place a heel lift under the right heel. Rest the left leg on the floor at a 90-degree angle. Hinge forward from the waist. Plant the large right toe on the ground and evenly balance the weight onto the ball of the right foot. Then, push into the ground with the right foot, leg, and buttocks to lift the left knee off the ground. All the weight will be in the right leg, and the left leg should be relaxed as it lifts. Lift only a few inches. Lower to the floor. Switch legs.

CORE REHABILITATION

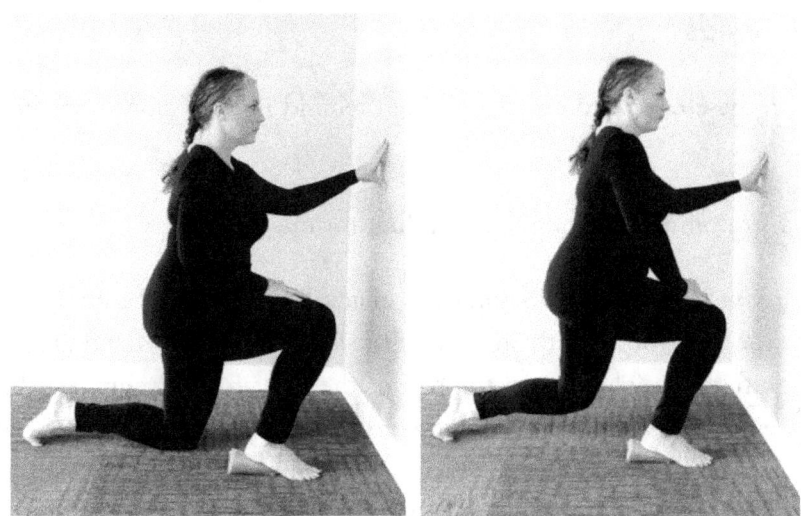

Figure 25. (*Left to right*) The model is in the initial position of single leg push-up. The model is in the fully engaged push-up position.

Knees Out

Notes: This exercise was one that Olivia assigned when I began complaining of my foot issues after I began running in 2022. Once I began these exercises, I realized how weak I was above the feet. I also developed an Achilles issue in my left ankle.

Execution: Stand with bare feet. Then place one foot a few inches behind you. Transition your weight from the front to the back by bending the front leg and straightening it. The goal in this exercise is for the arch to move as the leg bends and straightens. Repeat this motion several times on the same leg. Then switch legs. Repeat.

Calf Bends

Notes: These calf bend exercises helped rebuild my calf along with knees out.

Hint: I recommend lifting the back foot for the exercise.

Execution: Stand a few inches in front of a wall with the palms on the wall. Place the right foot slightly in front of the left foot. Slightly bend the front leg. Shift the weight toward the ball of the right foot. Evenly distribute the weight across the ball of the foot and anchor all the toes to the floor. Keep the hips centered, level, and facing the wall. Press into the outer right knee without bending it outwards. Press into the ground to verify the foot is evenly planted. Lift the back foot. Try to keep the muscles of the calf engaged while relaxing the shin muscles. Maintain the position of the body over the right foot and evenly distribute the weight. Hold.

When able, move backward using the calf muscle. After holding the pose, envision a rubber band pulling the calf muscle back to slightly straighten the leg. Keep the shin relaxed. Maintain even pressure of the ball of the foot on the floor at all times. Slightly press into the outer right knee. Keep the upper body and neck relaxed. Then, switch sides.

CORE REHABILITATION

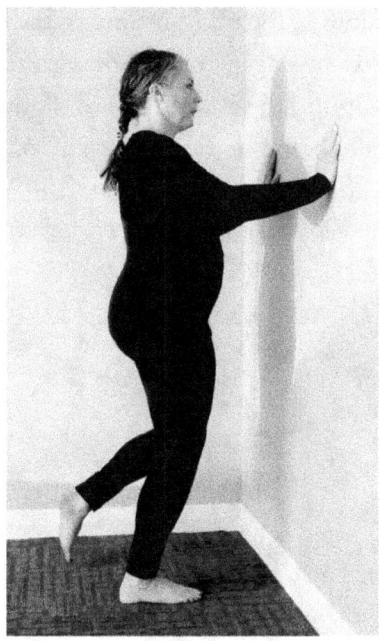

Figure 26. Calf bends.

Air Squat

Notes: I tried so many squat variations. I failed at all of them. I couldn't even correctly chair squat. Here is one version that seemed to finally work.

Weak hamstrings make it difficult to squat in appropriate form. To correct this, use something to elevate the heels, such as a slanted heel lift (as shown in Figure 27). When squatting, make sure to not break form. Examples include the back curling, the pelvis tucking under, or jutting out. Keep the upper body upright while visualizing the buttocks as close to the back of the legs as possible.

Execution: Stand with feet hip distance apart. Place the feet on lifts, if necessary. If able, hold the arms bent in front of the body. If not possible, the arms can hang at the sides of the body. Maintain the core. The abdominals and pelvic floor should stay engaged. Anchor with the big toes and evenly press the ball of the foot into the ground. Bend slightly at the knees. Then, hinge at the hips to tilt the upper body forward. Keep the back straight. Lower the legs and buttocks. Return to the starting position.

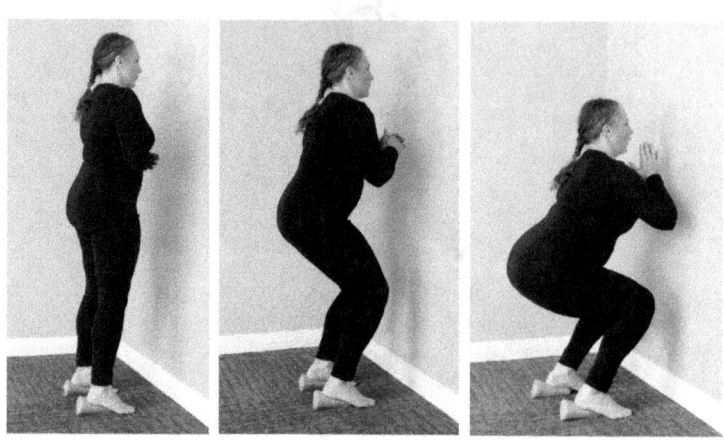

Figure 27. Various stages of air squat are shown.

Single Leg Static Lunge

Notes: This is one variation used to work toward the single leg lunge.

Hint: Lower as far as possible and hold the position. This may be only an inch. Use a balancing aid, such as a table or foam roller, to hold onto.

Dr. Craner's tip: Correctness of form is the highest priority at any time, but especially in a scenario like this where a patient is putting variations together to form a whole exercise.

When lowering, visualize the front leg muscles pulling toward the back wall and back leg muscles moving toward the front wall. However, in reality, they will remain stationary. It is only a visioning exercise to activate and engage the muscles.

Execution: Stand with the feet together. Then, move the right foot forward a few inches. Plant the big toe into the ground. Press into the ground with the ball of the foot, evenly. Extend the left leg behind the body. Place the toes of the left foot on the ground. Maintain the core. Bend the right leg at the knee to lower toward the ground. Simultaneously, bend the back leg. Return to the starting position. Switch legs.

EXERCISES TO AVOID

Side plank on knees

Notes: Side plank on knees is a great core exercise, and since it was on my knees, I thought it would be easy and safe. Eventually I noticed a problem after months of doing the exercise. This exercise resulted in worsening my facial spasms and TMJ issues. My neck and thoracic muscles were too weak to support myself on my elbow, even when my lower body was supported by a knee. The elbow support aggravated the nerves in my neck and face. It worsened my fascial spasms and TMJ issues. When I told Olivia, she had me stop doing them. As of 2024, I still avoid this exercise.

22.
NECK REHABILITATION

In addition to the cervical herniation, I also sustained whiplash from the accident. Dr. Murphy provided some insight into whiplash. He said the neck region includes the noodle-shaped body part we call a neck, as well as the soft tissue region of the upper back. The neck supports an 8-lb head. During a motor vehicle accident, the head whips back and forth on the neck like a bowling ball. This causes substantial damage to the muscles and ligaments of the cervical spine resulting in tears, strains and microtears. While microtears don't result in visible bruising, they are the reason it is so difficult to heal from whiplash. Even when these tears heal, the tissue heals as scar tissue instead of the previously healthy tissue. This new scar tissue results in a stiffer neck movement. Dr. Murphy taught me that in order to regain neck mobility, the scar tissue must be broken down.

Scar tissue is actually considered inflammation. Dr. Murphy highlighted the consequences of inflamed tissue supporting a bowling ball. With daily use, the scar tissue causes more inflammation. In addition, scar tissue can cause more scar tissue over time. Finally, it becomes difficult to isolate the neck muscles in order to strengthen them because they are holding a head the weight of a bowling ball. This combination of scar tissue and a "bowling ball" is why healing the muscles of the neck is a unique challenge.

Part of the reason why some core exercises worsened my facial spasms was because I was overcompensating for my weak core by using my neck muscles to perform the exercises. In addition, my neck muscles were already severely weakened from the whiplash. These muscles were constantly strained all day by holding a "bowling ball." The muscle imbalances began to appear over time as the muscles atrophied and healthier muscles began to compensate for the injured muscles. I was exacerbating the injured muscles in my neck by gritting my jaw and teeth. I was straining my neck muscles. In addition, I had the added concern of fascia injuries.

As the years passed, I had an instance where I sneezed and blew a vertebra out of alignment in my neck. This meant I had to hold my head to lie down. I could no longer support it. A quick chiropractic visit to Dr. Murphy was able to fix it, but my whiplashed muscles were so weak that something as insignificant as sneezing could have a negative impact. Thankfully, I don't have this problem any more. In fact, I endured what I called The Christmas Death Plague in 2022. I was testing negative for COVID but I lost my voice, had a fever, and coughed so hard that I thought I would be calling 911 to breathe again. I was coughing hard for 10-15 minute durations. I may have had a 60-second break between coughing spells at my worst. The coughing fits were so severe it tested my neck, but it held. I didn't have one vertebra slip out of position. It's these little things that I took for granted before the accident. I was excited to have proof I had strengthened my neck muscles with my rehabilitation plan.

In 2022, I could still pinpoint the exact location of the cervical spine injury even though I didn't have the radiating pain anymore. Even my massage therapists were able to feel a difference in the area. The best description to me was it felt like a rock. With continued strength training and functional rehabilitation, I hope to also heal this region. My goal is to never need surgery, despite the accident increasing my chances for needing surgery in this region. This is one reason why I work so hard to heal. I would like to die an old person without ever needing spine surgery. In 2023, I was feeling much better in this area. I hope it means the rehabilitation plan is working.

NECK REHABILITATION

The question of spine surgery brings me to an interesting thought. When I first had my accident, I was prepared for surgery. I wanted to heal and be better. I had this idea that surgery would be a quick fix. Now, I know surgery would not have healed me. Dr. Craner provided insight into chiropractic benefits after surgery. Once a person has spine surgery, there are often two successive surgeries. Post-surgery, joint movement changes movement of the spine. Scar tissue occurs around the surgical area, which can irritate the region. This irritation can result in future surgeries. Chiropractic adjustments would likely restore functional movement to the region in order to prevent future spinal surgeries, as well as decelerate degeneration.[1] This only made me want to work harder to heal my neck. The idea of needing multiple neck surgeries instead of one was horrifying. I am very thankful my spine surgeon chose rehabilitation over surgery.

I saw a lot of doctors the first year and was adamant about my facial and jaw pain. However, they weren't suggesting ways of healing those complaints. I knew the left side of my jaw had been socked during the accident, as it had been the most glaring pain in trauma. I was alarmed my doctors were not taking my pain seriously. When I transitioned to Dr. Murphy in 2019, he realized my jaw was dislocated. He did an adjustment. However, the pain and spasms continued. In 2021, I visited a specialist at the Cleveland Clinic who diagnosed me with hemifacial spasms. He also diagnosed me with a dislocated temporomandibular joint (TMJ) on my left side.

I was referred to a TMJ specialist in February 2022. The TMJ specialist diagnosed me with a severe neck disability as my mobility was extremely restricted. He suggested a night guard. He also informed me that once the dislocation occurred, it would always occur. He suggested additional therapies, but they were not covered by insurance. I was also concerned that physical therapy would worsen my condition and the therapies would ultimately be a waste of my money. I looked online for TMJ

PAIN WITH POISE

exercises. I found several that I tried.

I considered the suggested nightguard. However, I wanted to see what my chiropractors could do first. By this time, I was at Active Edge. My pain was very severe. I would mutter. I felt like I was being continually pounded in the head, and my mouth would draw on the left. The pain could also trigger trauma. In addition, this particular pain was more punishing than the other pain. There was something about this particular location that was a numbing, confusing, and gnawing pain. It was a different kind of pain. They did dry needling, adjustments, and monitored my exercises.

The hemifacial diagnosis was for the left side of my face. My spasms were so severe they would completely distort my face. One time, they caused a nosebleed. I was staring in the mirror when one happened. It looked like my eye was turned the wrong side out. It was really grotesque. Upon reading, I learned these spasms can be due to several reasons, but mine were likely due to a facial nerve injury. A hemifacial spasm is best known for distorting half of the face due to an irritation of a facial nerve.[2]

One symptom of these spasms is forced eye closure. This reminded me of when I was in the shower soon after the accident and my eyelids refused to rise for me when I wanted them to do so. I had to pry them open. Thankfully, I do not have these spasms all the time. With continued strengthening of my upper body and neck, massage, and with less stress, these spasms have decreased.

However, I now have extreme pain in my ear and clicking. It feels like I have bugs in my ear. The clicking in my ear, plus the ear pain, can make me feel like I am losing my sanity. For me, I have found hemipelagic spasms to have a pain level associated with them.

I am learning ways to alleviate the issues, including applying mindfulness breathing. When I feel things moving, I start focusing on balancing myself via proper breathing, focusing on my heart chakra, and smiling. Unfortunately, hemifacial spasms can cause mental health issues.

NECK REHABILITATION

Self-consciousness, anxiety, and depression are all issues that may arise from living with hemifacial spasms.[3] They did make me self-conscious. I didn't want people to think I was making faces at them. I didn't want people to think badly of me. I usually ran and hid when I felt a spasm coming.

I am now learning more about my spasms. To ease the hemifacial spasms, it was pivotal to eliminate stress. Essentially, stress was an allergy to me. It was like I needed an epinephrine injection for stress. When more upset or after a workout, I may spasm. I now know my neck can spasm only on the left side. I have isolated the event. However, I have learned to relax and, so far, the spasm will stop. This, sadly, is how I know stress can exacerbate the underlying condition. However, stress is not the problem or the underlying condition. There is no such thing as having emotion in half my neck or stress in half my neck. Unfortunately, physical disability exists. With time, I hope this continues to lessen.

With the awareness of having weak neck muscles, TMJ issues, and spasms, I decided the key was to rebuild the neck muscles. I knew my neck muscles had been destroyed by the tractor-trailer. The muscles in the front of my neck were shockingly weak. I knew I needed to reduce my stress. I knew I was clenching my teeth. I assumed the extreme pain and dealing with all the stress was showing up in my face as jaw tension. The chiropractors at Active Edge recognized my stress levels, and highlighted how stress can worsen neck, jaw, and facial pain. As I was trying to juggle so much with daily life, I was highly stressed. Plus, people were being really mean.

This region of my face proved very interesting. Some days, it didn't give me very many issues. Other days, it controlled me. Over time, I began noticing a connection with increased activity, such as runs or upper body exercises, exacerbating that region of my face. Even trying to stand with a good posture for an extended time would aggravate my neck and TMJ. Part of the issue was my weakened muscles and injured fascia. Part of the issue was I had nerve issues. To counter some of the

PAIN WITH POISE

issues, Olivia assigned some of the breathing techniques. These were the best ways to strengthen my core, enhance my posture, and build the muscles, even in my neck.

In 2023, one of my Cleveland Clinic neurologists wanted me to sit with perfect posture. He was trying to reduce the inflammation of my nerves in my face. This proved very challenging as my muscles were so weak and imbalanced. To do this, I had to focus on my breathing and focus on continued rehabilitation with deep tissue work.

In addition, one of my Cleveland Clinic neurologists prescribed physical therapy, specifically for a nerve. He wanted me to begin with five repetitions of the assigned exercise for my rehabilitation. He said if I woke up the day after performing the five exercises and I was experiencing pain, I was to rest. I was not allowed to continue the exercises until everything was no longer inflamed. There were different levels of inflamed pain. The first day I had tried what he showed me and it was like being on fire. This was what I was accustomed to. It was scream-worthy pain.

At this point, I really gave up. I didn't think it would work. However, my local neurologist wanted me to try it as well. I turned to Active Edge and said, "Do your thing." My chiropractic assistant Ana applied skin rolling to the chest. She also did some initial assessments where we learned my limitations. This was the first time we learned I couldn't "serve" anything. I was unable to reach my arms forward. It caused my fingers to go numb on my left hand. Until this assessment, I didn't even realize I was going numb in my left hand. After years of living in overall pain, a bit of numbness wasn't glaring to me. However, the numbness indicated a bigger issue, and Ana was able to use it to come up with an exercise.

Then, we tried some exercises and had to do several variations until we found one that worked best. However, I still had issues with it. I met with another of Active Edge's movement trainers. She did a lot of fascia work on me. This was when we realized my left bicep was riddled with knots. In fact, she could hear them as she worked them out. We stopped working on them when I started seeing stars. For the first time since the accident, somebody had finally found the source of a major dysfunction. I was relieved. I could take a lacrosse ball home and roll the area.

NECK REHABILITATION EXERCISES

Finger-Neck Strengthening

Notes: After weeks in physical therapy and with my pain only worsening, my physical therapists decided to eliminate my therapy exercises to only manipulating putty with my fingers. It was the first time I finally felt like I was working my neck muscles without increasing the pain. I was extremely challenged by the exercise. I noted how it was a struggle for my core. I was happy. It felt like I finally had a good match for my capabilities and injuries.

Execution: Take putty of various strength levels and play with it using the hands. Fold it. Knead it. Press it into the table. Then, do it with one hand and with individual fingers.

Giraffe Stretch

Notes: Ana recommended this exercise to strengthen my neck muscles. In this exercise, take special care to relax the front neck muscles when tightening the back muscles. Sometimes I place my fingers on the back of my neck to feel the muscles engage. This will be a very light muscle engagement.

Execution: Pull the crown of the head straight to the ceiling and stretch the neck away from the shoulders. Then, tighten the muscles in the back of the neck without pulling the chin inward or tightening the other neck muscles.

Dr. Craner's Tip: If the traps will not relax, bend the elbows to form a 90-degree arm position. A therapist may then apply gentle pressure straight downward toward the ground at the elbows. This can relieve the feeling of tightness in the traps and also help activate the deep neck flexors more efficiently.

Snow Angels on Foam Roller

Notes: One of my massage therapists recommended this exercise for my neck in 2021.

Execution: Lie with the spine on top of a foam roller. Straddle with legs bent on either side. Then, make sure all parts of the spine, including the neck, are flattened against the foam roller. Next, take the arms and move them up and down along the sides of the body like a snow angel.

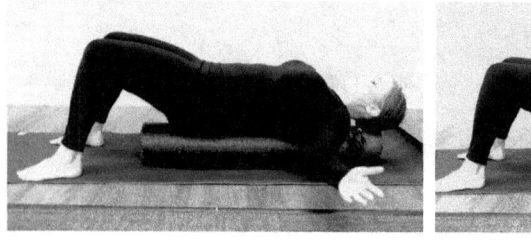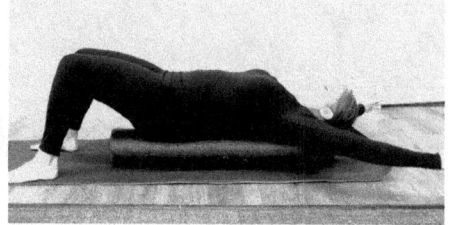

Figure 28. (*Left to right*) Starting position of the pose is shown; the model is performing full extension of snow angel.

Arm Wave on Foam Roller

Notes: My licensed massage therapist suggested this exercise to help with my tight muscles in my core and shoulders.

Execution: Lie on one side placing a foam roller under the rib cage close to the arm. Extend the lower arm over the foam roller. Then, move the arm up and down. It will look like a wave. Switch sides.

NECK REHABILITATION

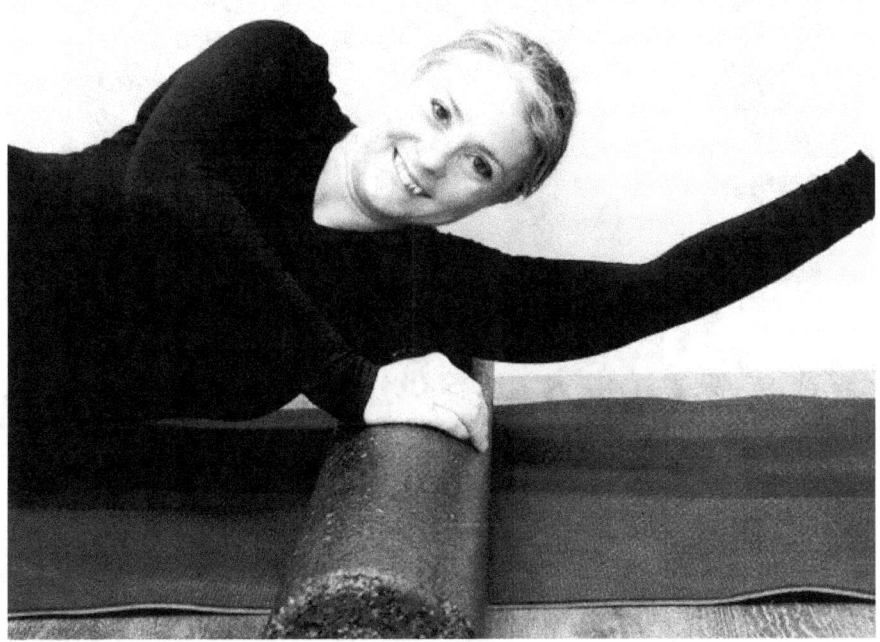

Figure 29. Arm wave on foam roller.

Arm Swing on Foam Roller

Notes: One of my massage therapists also suggested this exercise to help with my tight muscles through my core and shoulders.

Execution: Lie on one side. Then, place a foam roller under the lower rib cage close to the arm nearest to the floor. Extend the lower arm over the foam roller. Then, move the arm to the front of the foam roller. Rotate the arm along the floor to the opposite end of the foam roller. Continue the swinging motion.

PAIN WITH POISE

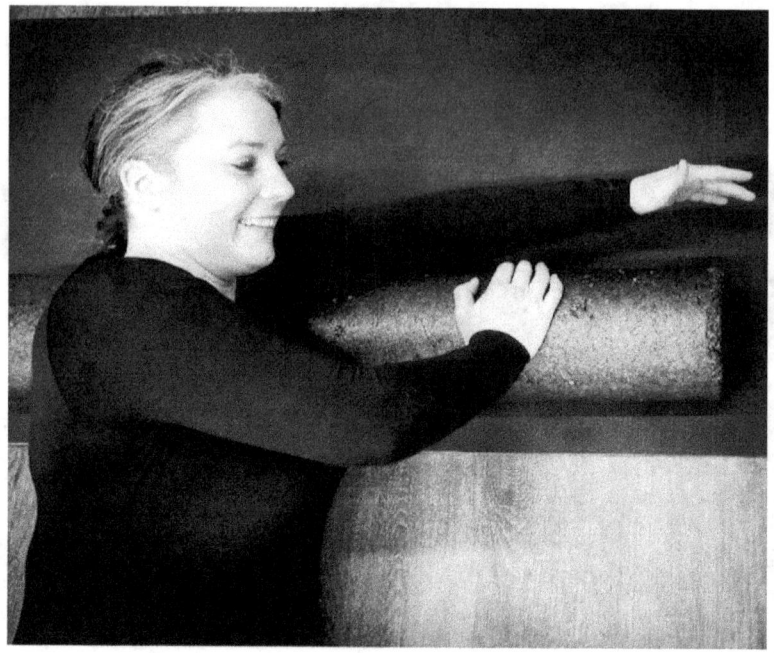

Figure 30. Arm swing on foam roller.

Towel Stretch

Notes: This exercise was suggested by Sybil, one of my licensed massage therapists, to help my tight shoulders. She suggested using a towel after a shower or even during a shower. I also liked using an exercise band. Maintaining an engaged core was my primary challenge.

Execution: Take a towel and lower it behind the head. Raise the towel back to the starting position. Make sure the core is engaged and does not extend outward during the exercise.

NECK REHABILITATION

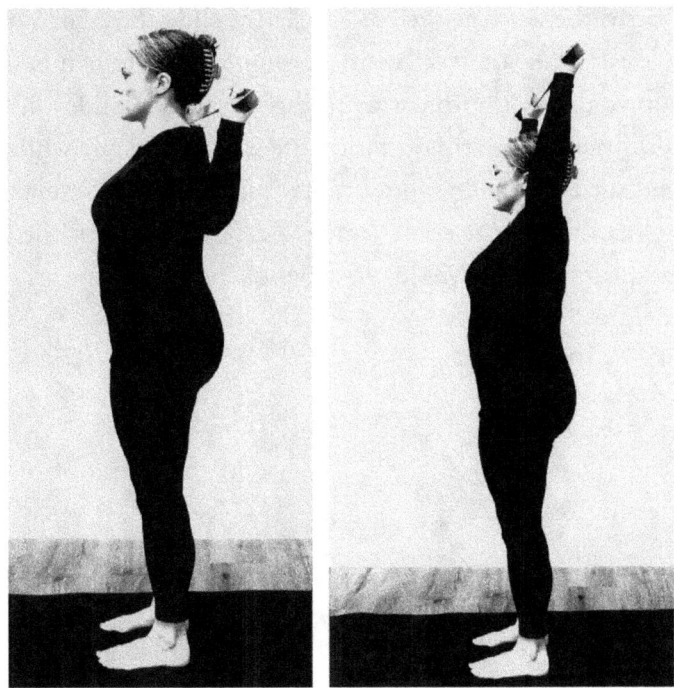

Figure 31. (*Left to right*) Starting position of towel stretch is shown; the model performing towel stretch.

Scapular Wall Slide

Notes: Searching for exercises to rebuild my thoracic region, I found one called a scapular wall slide with the exercise ball.[4] I adapted the exercise, because I eventually realized I couldn't use the exercise ball. Instead, I just leaned against the wall. Initially, I did have issues since my core was weak during this exercise. Once I applied breathing techniques 1 and 2, this became a more focused exercise as I was not having to fight my core. It also improved my flexibility.

Execution: Stand with the feet slightly away from the wall while the upper back and head rests against the wall. Keep the core engaged for the exercise. Bend the arms at the elbows. Then, slide the arms up the wall until the lower arms are level with the shoulders. The hands should be pointed upward and the forearms facing out. Then, slide the arms up the wall. Only slide the arms as far up the wall as possible while keeping the core engaged. The slide should come from the shoulder blade region, especially focusing on the spine region. Be careful to keep the neck and chin relaxed through the whole movement. Then, slide the arms back to the original position.

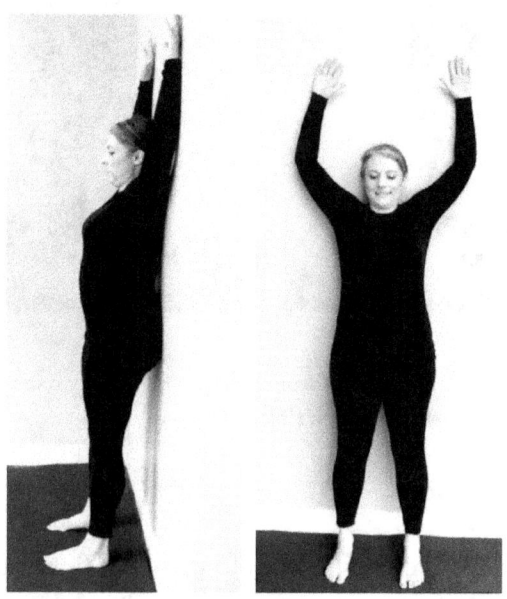

Figure 32. Scapular wall slide.

Variation 1: Wall Sit with Scapular Wall Slide

Notes: I had a great idea one day to combine the wall sit with the scapular wall slide. It was a great overall body workout that targeted all of my injured areas.

Execution: Stand with the feet a few inches away from a wall. If desired, place a small exercise ball between the knees. Plant the big toes on the floor. Maintain the core so the lower body and neck are flattened against the wall. Raise arms, keeping the core engaged so the lower arms are perpendicular to the shoulders and the upper arms are pointed upward. Slide the arms up the wall while sliding down the wall. Lower until in a chair position, if possible. Hold. Then, slide the arms back to the original position while returning to standing position. Repeat.

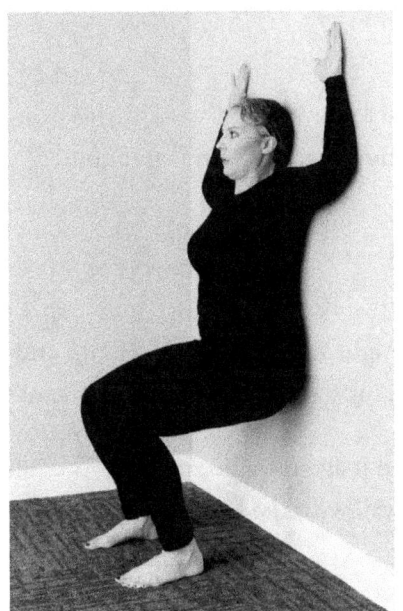 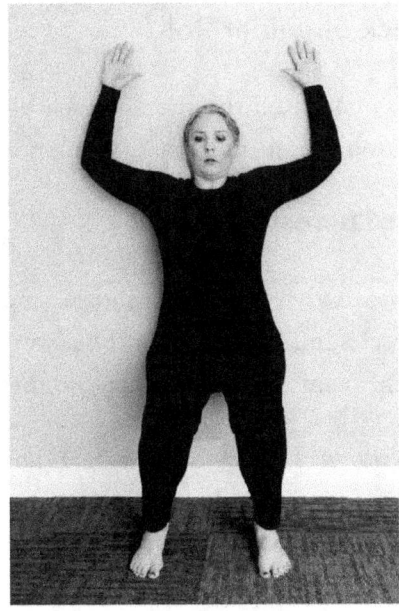

Figure 33. Various angles of wall sit with scapular wall slide.

Forward Shoulder Roll

Notes: The second physical therapy exercise I attempted to do post-accident was the forward shoulder roll. I could not do it. However, I could do it pre-accident with ease. There was nothing like sitting there in a chair and thinking "move, move, move" while nothing moved. It was terrifying.

However, I was advised to try a backward shoulder roll. That I could do. I was then introduced to what I would practice several times in therapy. If one direction would not work, I would need to try the opposite direction first. If that worked, I would then try the original direction. This exercise can be done standing or sitting.

Execution: Roll the shoulders forward, under, and toward the back of the room. Return to the starting position by doing a full rotation.

Back Shoulder Roll

Execution: Roll the shoulders backward, under, and toward the front of the room. Return to the starting position by doing a full rotation.

Pec Lacrosse Ball Roll

Notes: Active Edge's Ana showed me this exercise in order to release tight muscles in my pec region. I had very tight muscles in this region, and we spent many sessions working on these muscles to help them release.

Execution: Take a lacrosse ball and hold it against a pec muscle. Then, lean against a wall. Roll up and down the wall with the lacrosse ball. Repeat on the other side.

Prone Arm Raise

Notes: This was a successful variation of an exercise I had been assigned at Location 2.

Execution: Lie face down on the floor with the legs extended. Squeeze the glutes. Rest the forehead against the floor. Extend the arms at the shoulders so they are reaching to opposite sides of the room. Then, engage the muscles between the shoulder blades to lift the arms. This will prevent straining the muscles in the neck. Be careful to not tighten the jaw. Then, lower the arms back to the floor.

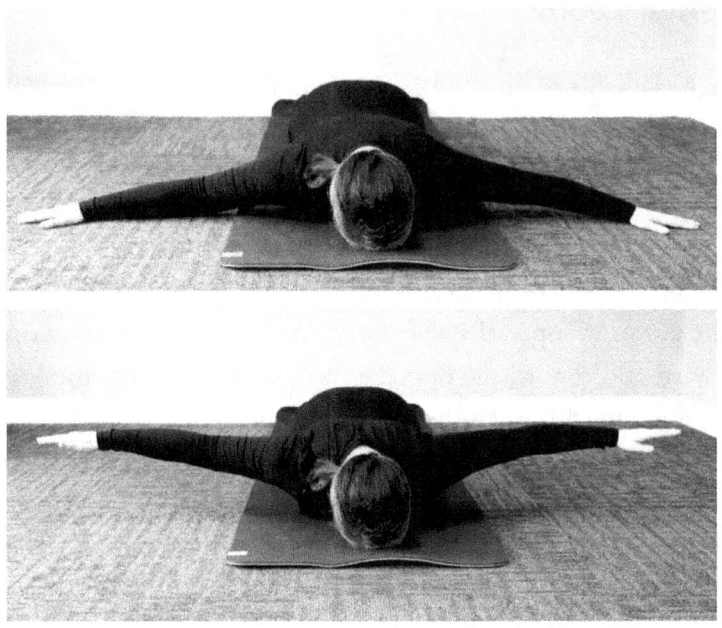

Figure 34 (*Top to bottom*) Starting position is shown; the full extension of prone lateral raise is shown.

Resisted Closing of the Mouth

Notes: Active Edge suggested this TMJ exercise, which was a great addition to the other TMJ exercises I was doing.

Execution: Open the mouth as wide as possible. Lightly place the fingers on the lower teeth. Then, slowly raise the lower jaw until the mouth is partly closed. Resist lightly with the fingers. Hold. Then, relax the mouth. Open the mouth as wide as possible a second time. Place the fingers on the lower teeth. When slowly raising the lower jaw part way, resist with more force using the fingers. Hold. Then, relax. Do this exercise twice.

Supported Cobra Stretch

Notes: I was unable to do a full cobra stretch with a back injury. However, this modification was a great way of stretching and building up to one as recommended at Active Edge. This was a very challenging exercise.

Execution: Lie on the ground with the elbows under the shoulders. To lift the upper body, begin extension from the cervical spine (neck), but keep the core and especially the lower abdomen engaged. Continue lifting upward and toward the opposite wall (away from the toes) with the cervical spine (neck). Keep the lower abdomen engaged and also curling upward so the spine curls as one. Think of lifting from the spine and not from the abdomen or back. The forearms are only used to provide even support but are not pushing the body upward. The upper body should be separating and lifting away from the forearms. Think of separating each vertebra on the lift. Using the upper body, apply pressure to the forearms to raise the upper body. Keep the chin level. Then, slowly lower back to the floor. Only raise as high as feels comfortable.

NECK REHABILITATION

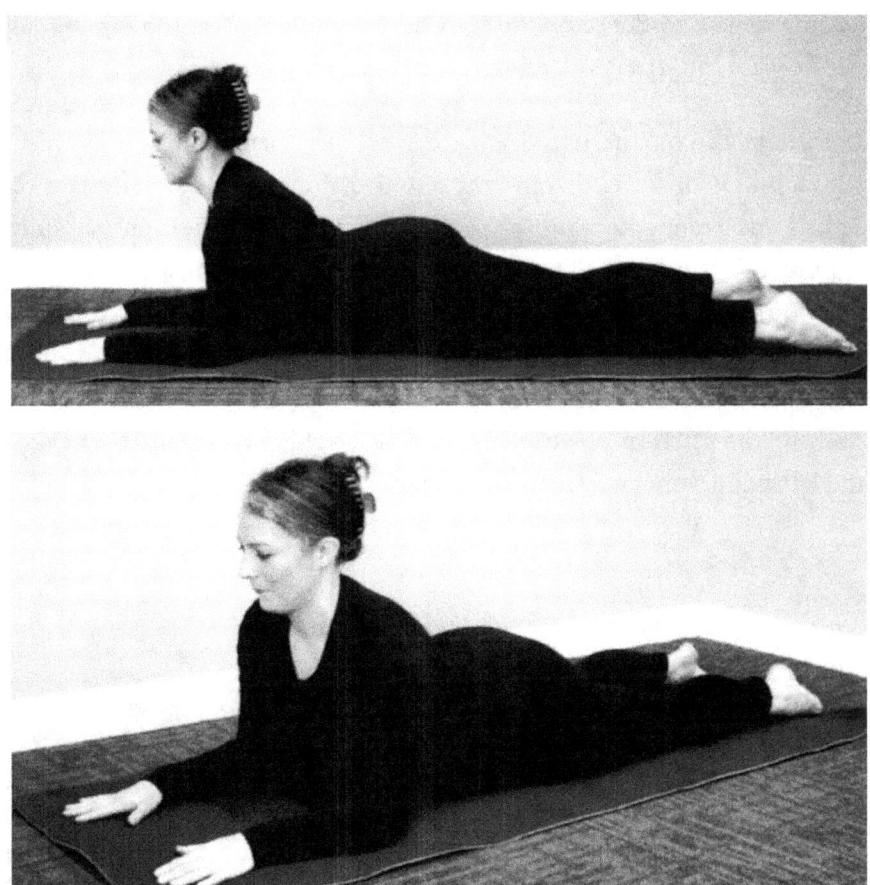

Figure 35. Various angles of the model performing supported cobra stretch at full extension.

Thoracic Windmill

Notes: This exercise was one of the very first exercises assigned at Location 2. However, it caused me pain. I finally tried it again at some point at least two years later with some modifications. I used a pillow or foam roller under my head. I even began supporting my upper back with a rolled towel. It's one I now consider an easy stretch. At the time, I had too much healing to go in order to do the exercise. My muscles were too injured, my nerves were too irritated, and my fascia was too damaged.

Execution: Lie on the left side with the knees bent. Support the neck with a pillow or towel. Extend the left arm along the floor and place the right arm extended on top of the left. Then, rotate the right shoulder behind the back and toward the floor. Bring the right arm along the body during the rotation and fully extend it to the right side of the body. The right fingers should point to the opposite side of the room from the left fingers. Return to the starting position by rotating the right shoulder back to the starting position. Extend the right fingers slightly beyond the left hand's fingers. Then, switch sides.

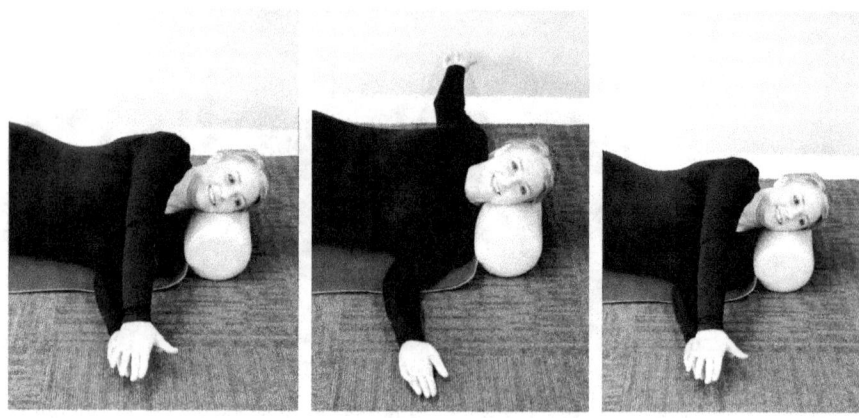

Figure 36. (*Left to right*) Various stages of thoracic windmill.

Wall Short Seated Reach

Notes: This is a nice stretch for the neck and shoulders. I could only do the forward stretch.

NECK REHABILITATION

Execution: Sit with the buttocks on the ground and the mid to low back flat against the wall. Let the legs extend straight on the floor in front of the body. Bend the knees one leg at a time and bring them as close to the chest as possible. Keep the knees together and feet slightly apart. During the exercise, do not let the legs rotate outward. Inhale through the nose. With the arms extended in front of the chest, exhale through the mouth and reach forward with the arms. The upper back and shoulders will move off the wall with the arms, while the lower back—from the bra line to the beltline—will stay against the wall. If necessary, rest the arms on the knees. Pause 3 seconds, if possible. Return to the starting position on the exhale.

Variation 1: After reaching the first full extension, maintain the position. Inhale through the nose and concentrate on breathing into the back of the chest wall without raising or tensing the shoulders. Exhale through the mouth, and reach farther with your arms, if possible. Then, return to the wall. Repeat.[5]

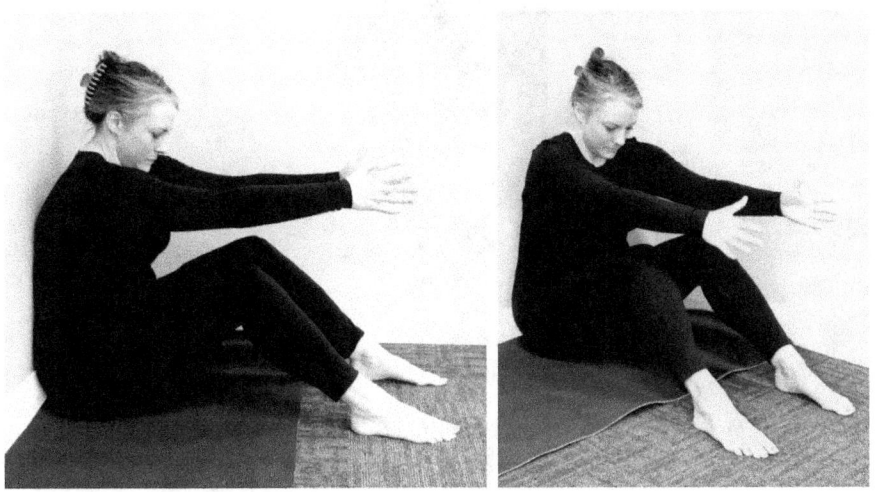

Figure 37. Various stages of wall short seated reach.

Door Stretch

Notes: This is a fantastic stretch for the neck, shoulders, and arms.

Execution: Stand in the opening of a door between the doorjamb. Bend the arms at the elbows and raise them to shoulder level. Place the palms against the doorjamb. Lean the body forward from the feet while keeping the feet, especially the heels, flat on the floor. Form a slight plank with the body but with arms to the side. Press the palms into the doorjamb. Do not press the arms against the door. Hold. Then, release.

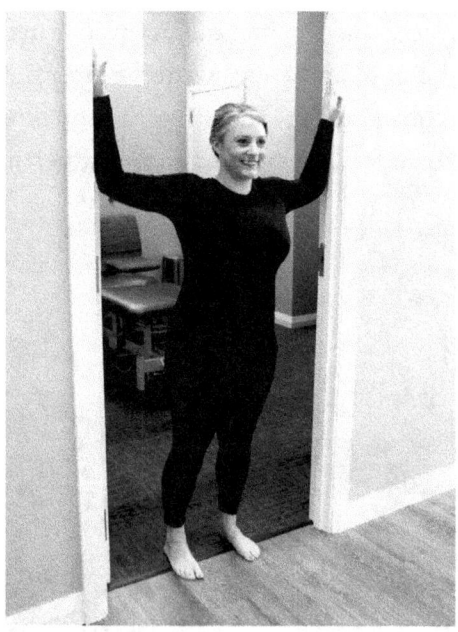

Figure 38. The model is extending the arms upward and into the door frame to perform door stretch.

NECK REHABILITATION

Lateral Flexion Stretch

Notes: This was the first stretch my spine surgeon's physician assistant recommended. If my spine had a fracture, the side-to-side motion of this stretch would have been safe. A forward and backward motion with chin to chest was not a safe motion for a broken spine. I found using a hand to increase the stretch increased inflammation, so I chose to not use a hand in my stretches. This stretch can be performed sitting or standing. Focus on breathing three-dimensionally. (See breathing techniques.)

Execution: Keep a straight spine with good posture. Inhale through the nose. Lean the head to the right shoulder without moving the shoulder upward. Hold. Exhale through the mouth while returning the head to the starting position. Repeat the stretch but lean the head to the left shoulder. Hold.

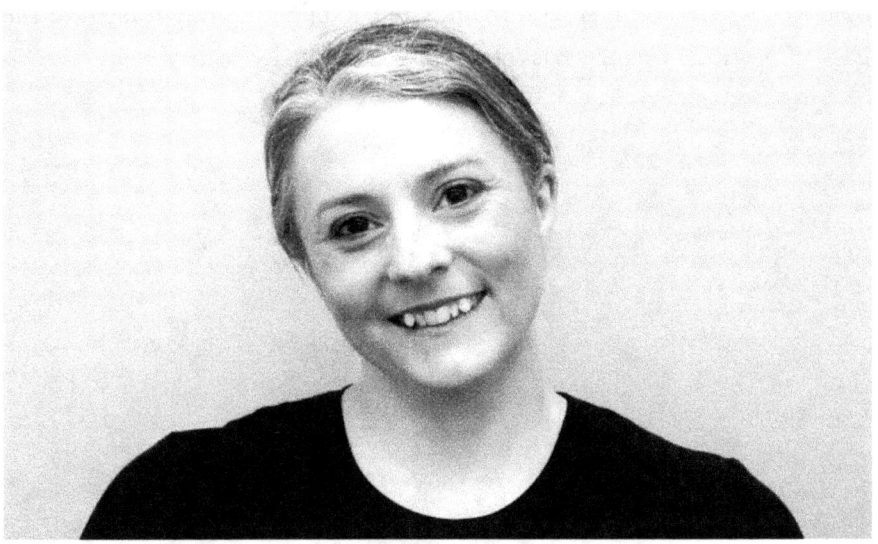

Figure 39. Lateral flexion stretch.

Opposite Side Face Arm Stretch

Notes: Ana, one of the chiropractic assistants at Active Edge, wanted to try opposite side face arm stretch as part of my physical therapy to resolve the irritated nerve in my left side. However, it irritated the nerve that was causing me issues. Here are a few variations that seemed to work well.

Tip: This exercise can be done standing or sitting. If sitting, extend the arm to the side and move the hand up and down at the wrist.

Execution: Stand with the feet hip width apart. Place the right arm against the wall at shoulder height. Keep the shoulder down. Turn the head to look to the left. If able, straighten the right arm. The hand should be pressed flat against the wall. Rotate the right hip a few degrees to the back, rotating the shoulder with it. Return to the starting position. Do a few rotations. Then, hold and stretch the arm with the hip and shoulder slightly rotated to the back, if possible. Change sides and repeat with the left arm.

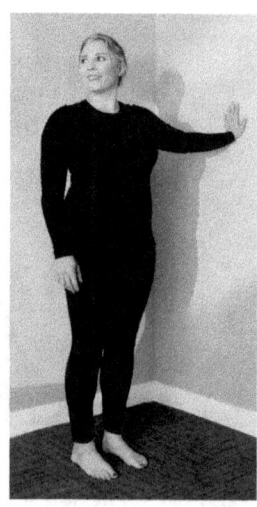

Figure 40. Opposite Side Face Arm Stretch.

NECK REHABILITATION

Variation 1: Same Side Face Arm Stretch

Execution: Stand with the feet hip width apart. Place the right arm against the wall at shoulder height. Keep the shoulder down. Turn the head to look to the right. If able, straighten the right arm. The hand should be pressed flat against the wall. Rotate the right hip a few degrees to the back, rotating the shoulder with it. Return to the starting position. Do a few rotations. Then, hold and stretch the arm with the hip and shoulder slightly rotated to the back, if possible. Change sides and repeat with the left arm.

Variation 2: Air Arm Stretch

Execution: Extend the right arm at shoulder level with the fingers pointed toward the wall, if possible. Extend the arm out of the shoulder joint. Without letting the hand touch a wall, turn the face to look at the hand. Move the hand up and down at the wrist. Lower the right arm. Repeat with the left arm.

Tricep Dips

Note: This exercise was a great exercise for rebuilding the neck muscles. It can be performed on a solid elevated surface, such as a firm chair or on a stair.

Execution: Sit on the edge of a chair. Place the heels of the hands on the edge of the chair. Then, move the body off the chair so the buttocks are now in front of the chair. The arms should be straight. Bend the arms at the elbow to lower the body in front of the chair. Do not bend the elbows more than 90 degrees. Raise the body back to start position.

PAIN WITH POISE

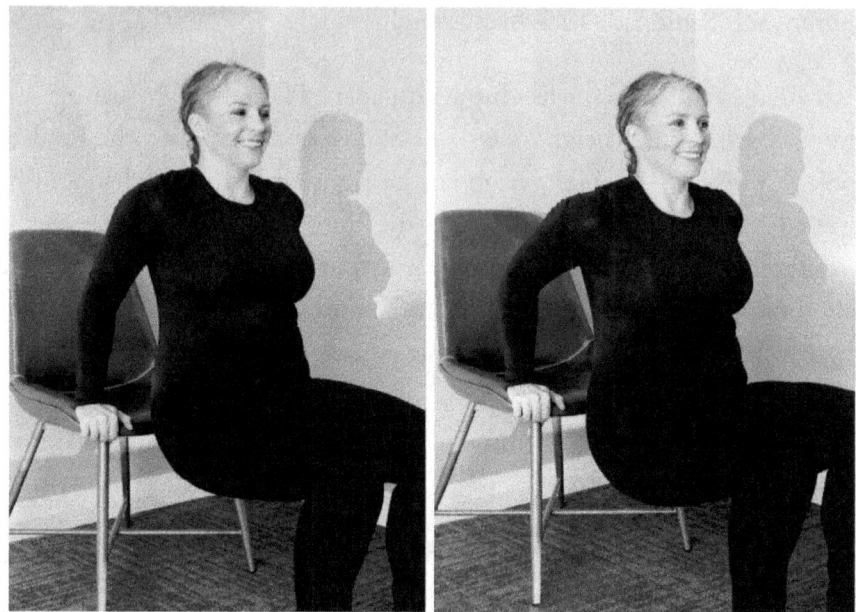

Figure 41. (*Left to right*) The model is in starting position of tricep dip. The model is dipping into tricep dip.

BUILDING TO A PUSH-UP

A push-up is normally considered a core and upper body exercise. However, I have it in the neck rehabilitation section as it aided in rebuilding my neck muscles as well as my core. We began with a wall push-up. Then, I improved to the incline push-up as I felt stronger. As my team learned more about my core and neck dysfunction, I would take breaks from the push-up or go back to the wall push-up.

One thing I found useful about this exercise was that it helped strengthen the muscles around my elbows. I had some irritation from the impact at my elbows. This even showed with an electromyography my neurologist performed. The electromyography indicated nerve irritability in my left elbow. Something was irritating my nerves. When I transitioned

NECK REHABILITATION

to an incline push-up, I began experiencing enough pain in my left elbow that I stopped doing push-ups. I mentioned this to Dr. Craner. I had done push-ups before the accident with no elbow issues.

Dr. Craner watched me do the incline push-ups. She suggested I rotate my elbows outward when I did my push-ups. I did, and it worked. The pain went away. This made me think about the power of POISE and being introspective. Another sprain, strain, etc. from the semi-truck that initially had been easily overlooked was yet again unveiled as I did my physical therapy.

Finally, the incline push-up highlighted my weak arms. I knew I had weak arms after the accident. Based on my injuries, I pieced together what happened to me during the accident since I had no memory of it. My best explanation was that my arms locked against the steering wheel and shoved my shoulder blades backward with incredible force when the 18-wheeler impacted my car. There was likely a torque as my car seat was swiveled inward. As the semi-trailer truck impacted the left back corner of my car seat, I had substantial damage to the left side of my upper back, and more injuries to the left side than right. This angled impact also caused the differences in my neck injuries.

While I have no memory of the accident, my nerves and brain have trauma memory and they remind me of actions, sensations, and feelings, which I also use to make sense of things. I still feel impacts and shudders and shakes which imitate a steering wheel shaking in my hands at an impact. Reversing the trauma damage was a combination of physical rehabilitation and allowing release of the emotions (and memories) from those body parts. Only then, could healing begin.

Wall Push-Up

Notes: Perform the wall push-up first before moving on to incline push-ups.

PAIN WITH POISE

Execution: Stand facing a wall with the feet a few inches away. Place the palms on the wall at shoulder height. Focus the eyes on the wall. During the duration of the push-up, keep the eyes focused on the same location. Engage the core and squeeze the glutes. Exhale into the abdomen. Lower the body toward the wall by bending at the elbows. Maintain the plank position as the chest moves toward the wall. On the inhale, begin straightening the arms. Slowly push away from the wall to return to the starting position.

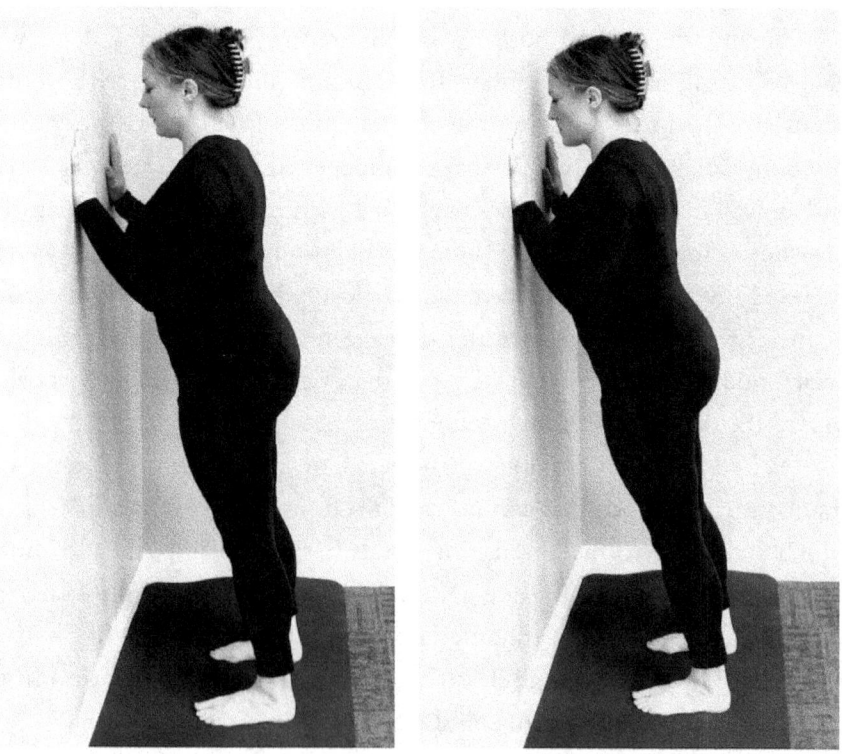

Figure 42. (*Left to right*) The model is in starting position; the model is engaged in a full wall push-up.

NECK REHABILITATION

Incline Push-Up

Notes: Perform the incline push-up after building strength with the wall push-up. Perform at various inclines, such as a counter, couch, etc. This exercise can be variable depending upon any flare-ups. On my strong days, I can do up to 10 incline push-ups. On my weak days, I can barely do 2 incline push-ups.

Tip: On weak days, a visit to the chiropractor may correct the dysfunction.

Execution: Stand facing an inclined surface. Place the palms on the top of the surface. Verify the elbows are rotated slightly outward. Focus the eyes on a spot slightly in front of the eyes' natural gaze. Hold the gaze at the same location for the whole exercise. Be careful to not tilt the head. Engage the core. On the exhale, bend at the elbows to lower the body toward the surface. Maintain the plank position as the chest lowers. On the inhale, begin straightening the arms. Slowly push away from the surface to return to the starting position.

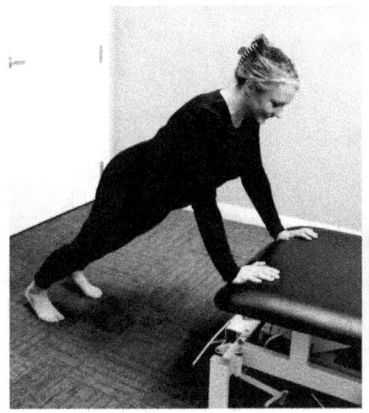
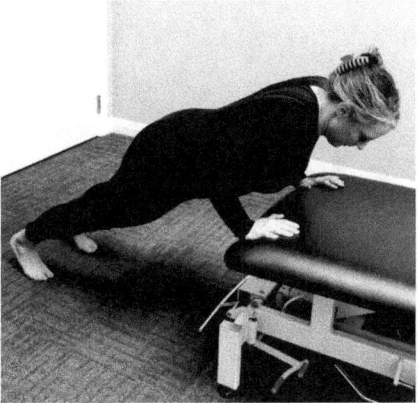

Figure 43. (*Left to right*) The model is in starting position of incline push-up; the model is performing incline push-up.

23.
WEIGHT REHABILITATION

Prior to the accident, I did a regular weight routine. I had my own free hand weights. I started lifting weights regularly beginning in graduate school. At the time of the accident, I used 5- and 10-pound free hand weights.

A few years after the accident, I tried some of the exercises from my normal weight routine with no weights. When I thought I could use some extra weight, I used soup cans for weights. Increasing to even 1-lb weights was too extreme of a change for me. Then, I gradually increased the weight to 1-lb weights. My goal was to continue increasing weight gradually. I recommend purchasing cheap floor-length mirrors to use at home to check one's form. I followed POISE. This was very slow progress.

For comparison, Location 3 had me use the weight machine for my lower body. It was far too early. This is a great example of how my injury was complicated, intricate, and extreme. It didn't appear extreme, but it was.

WEIGHT REHABILITATION EXERCISES

Military Press

Notes: Post tractor-trailer, I found it very difficult to maintain my core and to keep my right leg rotated correctly. I also had limited mobility in my neck and shoulder region. Therefore, I struggled to maintain proper form with this exercise. I decided to start by using my exercise ball and did a sitting variation of the military press. Once I did the breathing techniques and my body began to pull itself back together, I was able to better focus on proper form.

Execution: Sit on an exercise ball. Maintain the core. If using weight, hold the appropriate weight in each hand. Bend the arms at the elbow to form 90-degree angles. Raise the bent arms to shoulder height so the hands are facing the ceiling. To correct the neck, use the giraffe stretch for proper placement. Then, slowly straighten the arms using the muscles of the upper back and shoulder blade region. Be careful not to disengage from the back to use only the upper neck muscles or to overcompensate with the jaw and front neck muscles. Slowly return to the starting position.

Lateral Raises

Notes: I had the same concerns with the lateral raises as I did with the military press. I was able to resolve them with the same corrections. I also began my lateral raise rehabilitation by sitting on the exercise ball.

Execution: Sit on an exercise ball. Maintain the core. If using weight, hold the appropriate weight in each hand. To correct the neck, use the giraffe stretch for proper placement. Hold both arms to the side of the body. Then, slowly raise both arms with palms facing down using the muscles of the upper back and shoulder blade region while being careful not to overcompensate using the back to use only the upper neck, front neck, or jaw muscles. Raise the arms as close to shoulder height as possible. Keep the arms as straight as possible. Slowly return to the starting position.

Palms Back Raises

Notes: I had the same concerns with the palms back raises as I did with the military press. I was able to resolve them with the same corrections. I also began my palms back raise rehabilitation by sitting on the exercise ball.

WEIGHT REHABILITATION

Execution: Sit on an exercise ball. Maintain the core. If using weight, hold the appropriate weight in each hand. To correct the neck, use the giraffe stretch for proper placement. Hold both arms to the side of the body. Then, raise both arms, straight, to the front of the body, with palms down. Use the muscles of the upper back, shoulder blades, and chest region while being careful not to overcompensate with the upper neck, front neck, and jaw muscles. Raise the arms as close to shoulder height as possible. Keep the arms as straight as possible. Slowly return to the starting position.

Upright Row

Notes: Before the accident, I loved the upright row. After the semi-trailer truck I had the same concerns with the upright row as I did with the military press. I was able to resolve them with the same corrections. I also began my upright row rehabilitation by sitting on the exercise ball.

Execution: Sit on an exercise ball. Maintain the core. If using weight, hold the appropriate weight in each hand. To correct the neck, use the giraffe stretch for proper placement. Hold both arms to the side front of the body. Then, bend the arms at the elbows. Leading with the elbows, bring the weights in front of the chest. Keep the arms and weight close to the torso for the whole movement. Use the muscles of the upper back and shoulder blade region while being careful not to overcompensate with the upper neck, front neck, and jaw muscles. Raise the elbows as close to shoulder height, if possible. However, maintain the elbows level with the hands.

Hint: Don't point the elbows to the ceiling and the arms to the floor. Slowly return to the starting position.

Front Raises

Notes: I also began my front raise rehabilitation by sitting on the exercise ball.

Execution: Sit on an exercise ball. Maintain the core. If using weight, hold the appropriate weight in each hand. To correct the neck, use the giraffe stretch for proper placement. Hold both arms to the sides of the body. Then, raise both arms, straight, in front of the body, with palms up. Use the muscles of the upper back and shoulder blade region while being careful not to overcompensate with the upper neck, front neck, and jaw muscles. Raise the arms as close to shoulder height as possible. Keep the arms as straight as possible. Slowly return to the starting position.

Dumbbell Kickback

Notes: Find a low surface to rest a knee on to perform the exercise. Another option is to sit on a chair or exercise ball.

Execution: Sit on an exercise ball. Lean slightly over at the hips keeping the full buttocks planted on the exercise ball. Keep a straight spine pulling out of the hips. Maintain the core. If using weight, hold the appropriate weight in each hand. To correct the neck, use the giraffe pose for proper placement. Hang both arms to the sides of the body. On the exhale, extend both arms slightly behind the body. Do not overcompensate with the upper neck, front of neck, and jaw muscles. Slowly return to the starting position.

Overhead Extension

Notes: Sit on an exercise ball or stand, if desired.

Execution: Sit on an exercise ball. Maintain the core. If using weight, hold the appropriate weight in the right hand. To correct the neck, use the giraffe stretch for proper placement. Extend the right arm toward the ceiling. Drop the shoulder. Bend at the elbow so the hand lowers behind the head. Only lower as far as possible. Slowly return to the starting position. Switch sides.

Alternating Curls

Notes: Alternating curls was an exercise I also used to love. However, as they involved cross-body movement and balancing, I realized something was wrong when I tried doing them while rehabbing. However, after applying the breathing techniques, this exercise became easier.

Execution: Sit on an exercise ball. Maintain the core. Hold the appropriate weight in each hand. To correct the neck, use the giraffe pose for proper placement. Hold both arms to the sides of the body. Then, bend one arm and raise the weight to waist height. The palm will be up. Use the muscles of the upper back and shoulder blade region while being careful not to disengage from the back to use only the upper neck muscles. Slowly return to the starting position. Repeat.

Curls

Notes: These can be done on the exercise ball or standing.

Execution: Maintain the core. Hold the appropriate weight in each hand. Hold both arms to the side of the body. Then, bend one arm and raise the weight to waist height. The palm will be up. Slowly return to the starting position. Repeat.

24.
LOWER BODY REHABILITATION

I didn't receive any rehabilitation for my lower body until 2019. This was not for lack of complaining. I told my doctors about it from the very beginning. When I looked down, my right leg looked twisted 45 degrees from my pelvis. The right side of my pelvis felt split and torn. Every visit, I highlighted these issues to them. I don't know if their medical textbooks had anything to prepare them for "right leg twisted 45 degrees," but I was livid. I felt diminished. I despised doctors.

I finally found a family physician who listened to me and sent me to physical therapy for my buttocks and leg injuries. I had groin injuries, and the pain was partly from a femoral nerve. In addition, that groin pain extended to only half my pelvis. It was my right side and stopped exactly mid-line. It extended inward, internally, and upward. Thankfully, by 2019, that inward pelvic pain was gone. I was very angry at those doctors, because that was very real pain.

While I worked with my physical therapist, I knew things just didn't feel right. It wasn't healing right. While some things were improving, it just felt off. When I applied the breathing techniques, I realized my issues were core related. However, along the way, I still had other areas of the legs and feet to rehab.

LOWER BODY REHABILITATION EXERCISES

Alphabet

Notes: I did this exercise as a runner. It's easy and something a person on bed rest is able to do. It's also great if one is ordered to not move their spine. Since the neck is connected to the feet, it's a good exercise to do for the neck, too.

Execution: Either standing or sitting, raise one foot. Then spell the alphabet with the foot from A to Z. Capital or lowercase letters can be used. Repeat with the other foot.

Spread Toes

Notes: This exercise was painful for me. I didn't do it until 2022 when I was starting to pull everything back together and noticed an issue with my feet. Olivia suggested this exercise. She said it was supposed to be easy. It was not, which signified I had an underlying issue. In fact, the first time I did it with my right foot, it triggered trauma from the semi-trailer truck. The left foot did not produce the same reaction. My right foot had some trauma memory.

Execution: Put the left hand's fingers between each toe of the right foot. Then, place the right hand over the top of the right foot. Hold the foot in place with the right foot. With the left fingers, rotate the toes from side to side. Repeat this movement 10-20 times. Then, move the toes back and forth 10-20 times. Switch feet.

LOWER BODY REHABILITATION

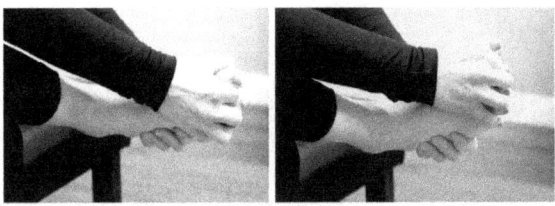

Figure 44. (*Left to right*) The model is in starting position of spread toes; the model is rotating the foot up.

Short Foot

Notes: This exercise was one of the first exercises I did with Olivia. She explained it would help my dysfunction in the pelvis region.

Execution: Pull the pants up to expose the ankles. Then, place the soles of both feet against the wall. Activate the small portion of the inner arch as if it is pulling the big toe toward the heel. Be careful to not engage the ankle muscles or other foot muscles. Do one foot or both feet together.

Knees Out

Notes: This exercise was one Olivia assigned when I began complaining of my foot issues after I began running in 2022. Once I began these exercises, I realized how weak I was above the feet. I also developed an Achilles issue in my left ankle.

Execution: Stand with bare feet. Then place one foot a few inches behind the body. Transition weight from the front to the back of the body by bending the front leg and straightening it. The goal in this exercise is for the arch to move as the leg bends and straightens. Repeat this motion several times on the same leg. Then, switch legs. Repeat.

Hamstring Curl

Notes: At first, when I was assigned this exercise in 2019, I was not using the right muscles. My buttocks were too injured, and my lower buttocks were atrophied. My pelvis was still too injured. When I did a hamstring curl, I really wasn't sure which muscle I was engaging, but I knew I was missing a lot of muscles. After applying the breathing techniques, 10-degree therapy, and squats, I could do a hamstring curl more efficiently.

Execution: Stand behind a couch. Place an object like a foam roller a few inches behind the couch. Step in front of the foam roller. Raise one leg and lower and tap the foot behind the foam roller. Raise the leg. Lower it and tap it behind the foam roller. Repeat. Switch legs.

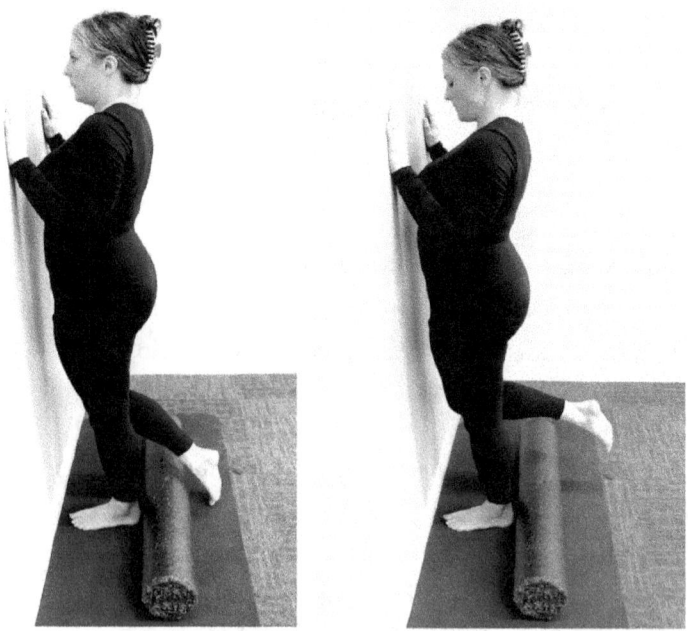

Figure 45. (Left to right) The model is in starting position of hamstring curl; the model is lifting the right foot up.

LOWER BODY REHABILITATION

Grapevine

Notes: I tried doing the grapevine in 2019. I used to do this all the time in my dance DVDs or at the gym in my dance classes. Then, the grapevine was easy. Now, I lacked the core strength along with all my head-to-toe injuries to call this move easy. The movement was stiff and I lacked bounce. I could not twist or wiggle. I highly recommend physical therapists incorporate this exercise into treatments.

Execution: Stand with the feet hip width apart. Step the left foot behind the right foot. Step the right foot to the side. Repeat. Continue this sidestep for the number of reps desired. Then, to reverse directions, step the right leg behind the left leg. Step the left leg to the side. Continue until back to the starting position.

Forward Fold Calf Raises

Notes: I had a major core dysfunction. I wanted to run again. I wanted to wear heels again. I needed calf muscles. Calf raises required a person to be upright. However, when I tried calf raises, I couldn't do them because of my core dysfunction. I found forward fold calf raises were a nice alternative. Once I did the breathing techniques and began to totally revamp my body, I was able to start doing calf raises again.

Execution: Find a staircase or just a chair or sofa. Bend over to place the hands on the surface. Then, raise onto the toes. To do this exercise, focus on using the legs and hips instead of the back muscles as the pivot location. Lower to the starting position. Repeat.

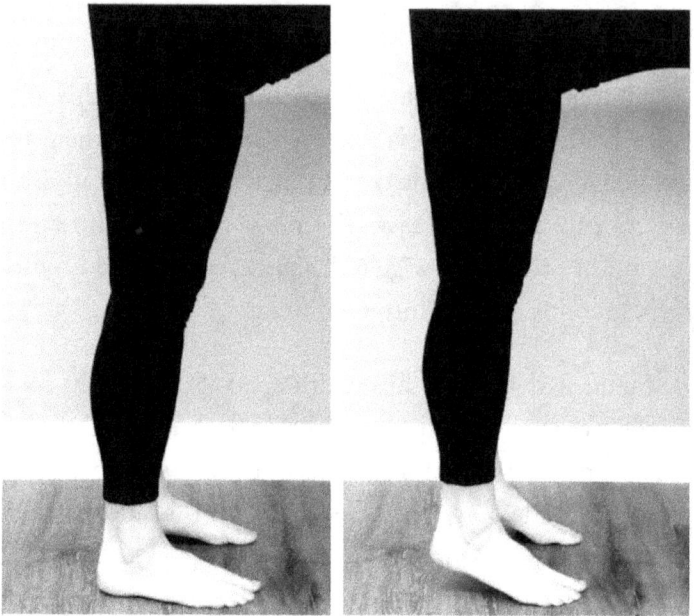

Figure 46. (*Left to right*) The starting position is shown; the model is performing a forward fold calf raise.

Reverse Toe Curl

Notes: This is an easy exercise one can do sitting or standing.

Execution: Take one foot and place it on the ground so the toes are curled under. Then, rotate the leg back and forth so the foot fully rotates from pinky toe to large toe and back. Repeat. Then, switch legs.

LOWER BODY REHABILITATION

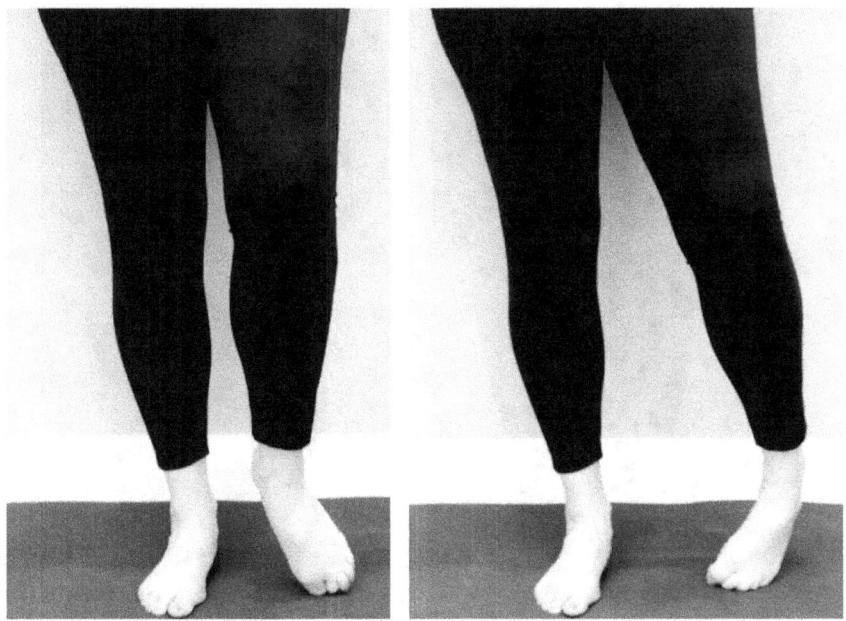

Figure 47. The model is rotating her foot back and forth to flex her curled toes for reverse toe curl.

Seated Calf Raises

Notes: This is a simple exercise one can do sitting. When possible, place a weight on the top of the legs to add resistance.

Execution: Sit in a chair with the back straight and core engaged. Raise onto the toes. Lower to the starting position. Repeat.

PAIN WITH POISE

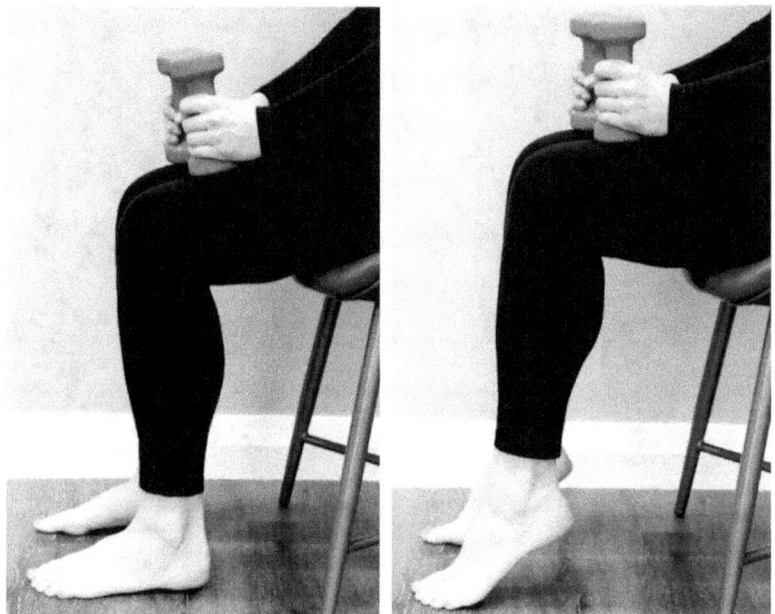

Figure 48. (*Left to right*) The starting position of the stretch is shown; the model is fully engaged in seated calf raise.

The Square

Notes: I used a foam roller for balance. Use an exercise band of appropriate resistance with one side looped around a table or chair that won't move. Don't allow slack in the band.

Execution: **Point 1**. Stand facing the band and loop. Loop the right foot in an exercise band. Slightly bend the left knee. Plant the ball of the left foot evenly into the ground. Balance on the left foot. Squeeze the buttocks. While squeezing the buttocks, move the right leg backward. Move the right leg forward to return to the starting position. Be careful to use the engaged buttocks to assist the leg instead of the lower back muscles. Do not use the hip flexors and let the buttocks relax.

LOWER BODY REHABILITATION

Point 2. Rotate 90 degrees to the left. Slightly bend the left knee. Plant the ball of the left foot evenly into the ground. Balance on the left foot. Squeeze the buttocks. While squeezing the buttocks, squeeze the right leg inward toward the left leg. Then, move the leg outward to the starting position. Be careful to use the engaged buttocks to assist the leg instead of the lower back muscles. Do not use the hip flexors and let the buttocks relax.

Point 3. Rotate 90 degrees to the left. Slightly bend the left knee. Plant the ball of the left foot evenly into the ground. Balance on the left foot. Squeeze the buttocks. While squeezing the buttocks, move the right leg forward. Be careful to use the engaged buttocks to assist the leg instead of the lower back muscles. Do not use the hip flexors and let the buttocks relax.

Point 4. Rotate 90 degrees to the left. Plant the ball of the left foot evenly into the ground. Balance on the left foot. Squeeze the buttocks. While squeezing the buttocks, cross the right leg in front of the left standing leg. Then, move the right leg back to the starting position. Be careful to use the engaged buttocks to assist the leg instead of the lower back muscles. Do not use the hip flexors and let the buttocks relax.

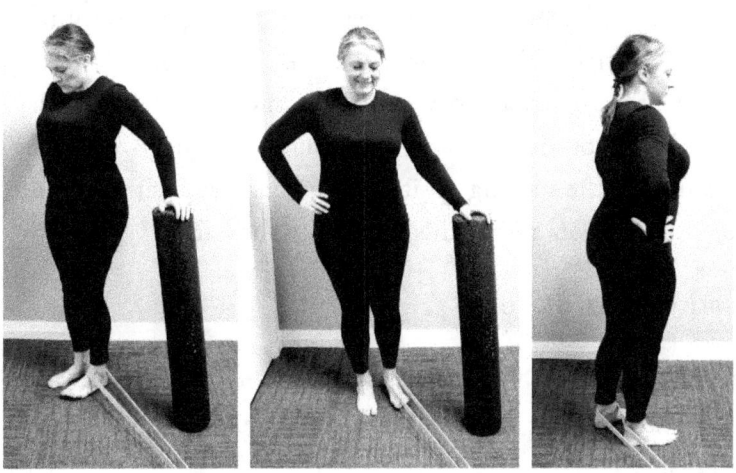

Figure 49. Various stages of the square are shown.

Heel Walks

Notes: I began incorporating heel walks to rebuild the buttocks and hamstrings. It worked better than anything else.

Execution: Stand upright. Begin walking with one foot in front of the other. Land on the heel of the front foot keeping the toes in the air. Then, lift the back foot to walk forward and land on the heel. The toes will be in the air. Repeat walking forward.

Lateral Forward Step

Notes: This is a great, easy exercise to begin for the lower body that involves balance, coordination, and cross-body involvement.

Execution: Stand with feet at hip distance. Move the right foot forward. Then, move the left foot forward. Then, move the right foot backward but to the right, as on the diagonal. Move the left foot back, on the diagonal, to return to the starting position. This starting position is shifted one step to the right. Then, repeat this exercise to the right. Continue moving sideways to the right. Then, reverse to the left. Move the left foot forward. Then, move the right foot forward. Then, move the left foot backward, but to the left, as on the diagonal. Move the right foot back, on the diagonal, to return to the starting position. This starting position is shifted one step to the left. Then, repeat this exercise to the left.

Banded Forward Step

Notes: Loop an exercise band of appropriate resistance above the knees. Be careful to not move the hips when walking. The hips should stay in a straight plane.

LOWER BODY REHABILITATION

Execution: Stand with feet at hip distance. Move the right foot forward. Then, move the left foot forward. Then, move the right foot forward again. Continue moving forward. Then, reverse. Return to start.

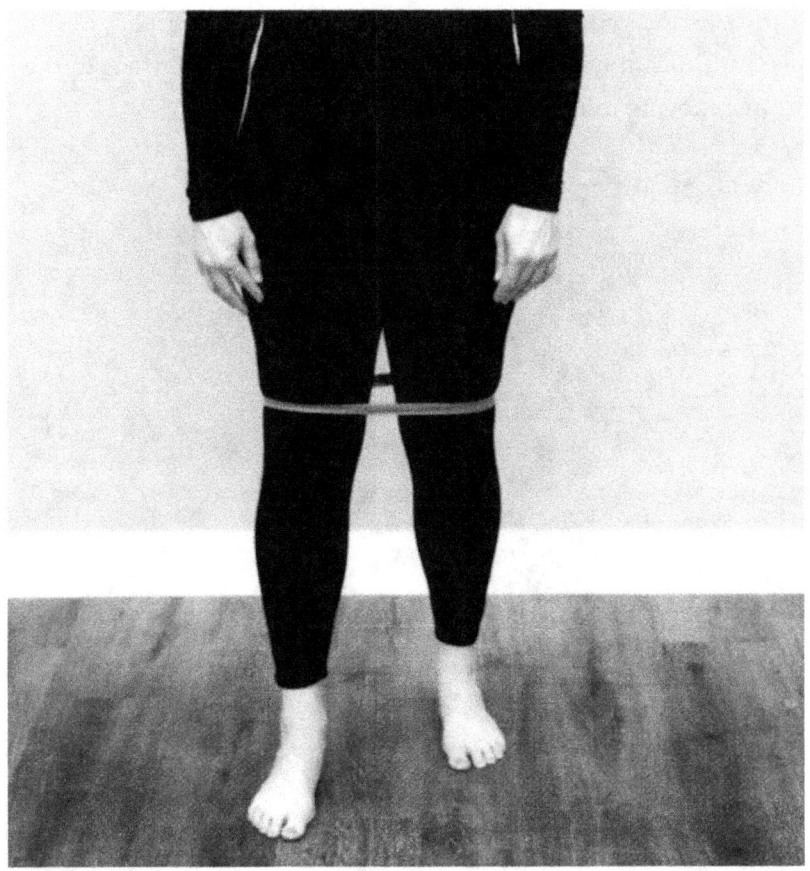

Figure 50. Banded forward step.

Banded Lateral Step

Notes: Loop an exercise band of appropriate resistance above the knees.

Execution: Stand with feet at hip distance. Move the right foot to the right. Continue moving to the right. Then, move the left foot to the left. Continue moving to the left. Return to start.

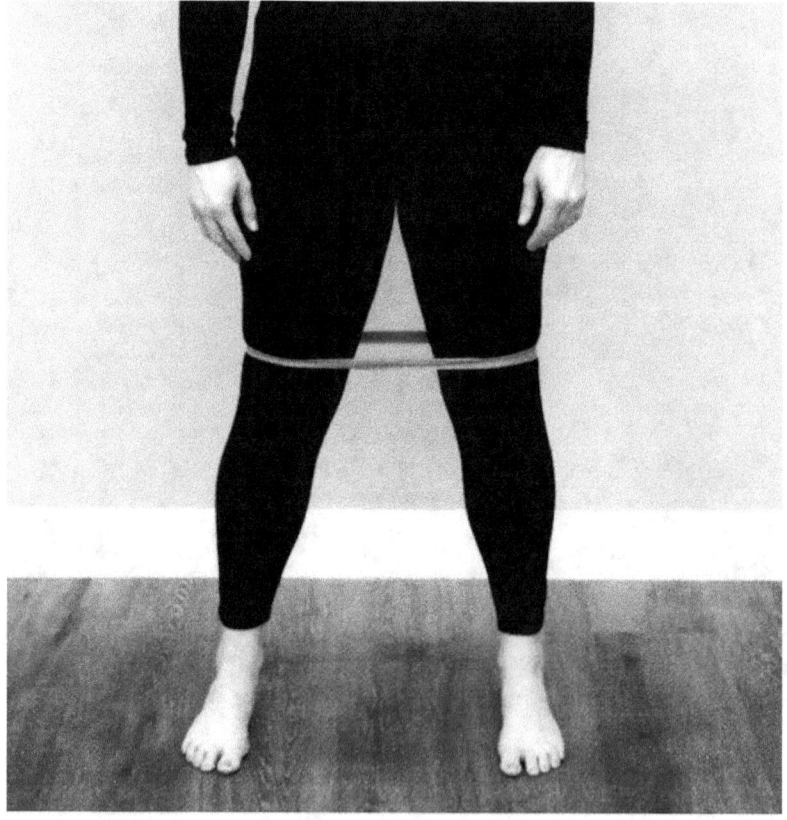

Figure 51. Banded lateral step.

LOWER BODY REHABILITATION

Glute Raises

Notes: For me, the worst of my lower body in physical therapy rehabilitation was my glutes. The first time I was assigned glute raises, I was unable to do them. I had no ability to activate the glute. I could use the back, the hamstrings, the hips, etc., but not the glutes. This was the region of my body after the accident that my brain informed me was set well in front of my body. Then upon returning to its normal location in my brain, I had no feeling in the bottom of my buttocks.

I was told to lift my leg. I could not. I literally could not. It was horrible. My physical therapist said to try harder. In order to lift my leg, I had to visualize my glute and focus so hard, I actually broke out into a sweat to lift my leg once. I used all my might. I think I did it a couple of times and I was unable to do any more. I went home mentally exhausted. However, over time, the feeling returned to my numb buttocks. My physical therapist was right. It was just atrophied muscle. My theory was my legs extended from the pelvis at impact. I had atrophied buttocks from a single impact.

When I went to the chiropractor, I got tweaks to the exercise as well as adjustments. The chiropractic, pelvic, and other adjustments made the exercise easier. In fact, there was also a neck connection which made my glute raises difficult. I was advised not to use my back in the lift of the glute raise. I continued to have adjustments over the next months to continue all the adjustments as I progressed.

Execution: Lie on the ground face down. Without engaging the back muscles, and using the glutes, lift the right leg. Lower the right leg. Lift the left leg. Lower the left leg. Repeat.

EXERCISES TO AVOID

The Static Quad Stretch

Many physical therapists recommended this stretch. However, this static exercise was insufficient for me. Instead, look for dynamic stretch alternatives.

25.
BALANCE REHABILITATION

Daily living is made easier due to balance. When humans execute an activity, they may place objects in a bag, transition from different surfaces while walking, or slip on a wet floor. Regardless of what activity the human performs, the body uses what is known as proprioception to stay safe. The body will sense the extra weight in the bag and adjust so the body won't tip over. The body will recognize a new surface and adjust to acclimate to the new surface. The body will rush into action when it detects a slip to protect itself and to stay upright. These are all ways the body uses proprioception to stay balanced.[1]

When the body is injured, proprioception can worsen, which increases one's risk for injury.[2] After the accident, my risk for injury did indeed greatly increase. My coordination and reaction time decreased greatly. If I stumbled, I couldn't catch myself. I just knew I was going down. I had two very hard falls during my recovery, and both times I fell awkwardly. I fell completely sideways as I was unable to bend anything. To prevent injury and falls, I simply altered my living. I moved slowly and became extremely cautious. I learned to not jump to help people but to do things at my pace. I moved in preparation to prevent people from touching me as they did not know how quickly they could cause pain.

I did several variations of balance exercises with physical therapists. However, I personally don't believe they were very useful until they were paired with the breathing techniques. In 2018, I remember my physical therapists commenting on how great my balance was while I was getting internally more and more upset with them. I knew how I felt before the accident when I balanced during yoga. I knew the difference in my body when I balanced after the crash, even if it superficially appeared I was great at balancing.

I continued doing balance exercises of some variation through the next few years. However, what was missing was finding the right combination of exercises to get my core to work together as one unit where all the pieces and parts were activating and functioning as one. I even did exercises on the balance board in physical therapy. While I loved the balance board exercises, they weren't fixing what was wrong.

In late 2020, I went to a family wedding. It was outside with a dance floor on the ground. I had to slide my feet to walk on it in flat riding boots to stay upright. Each bounce of the floor was enough to send me to my butt if I had picked my feet up off the floor to walk normally. It was even shocking to me. I was too uncoordinated. I was too unbalanced. I had no core. At this point, I seriously considered if I would ever recover. I had been in physical therapy for two years, and it wasn't working.

What could be wrong? Ultimately, my core was too dysfunctional for balance exercises. Even standing in place, my body was not in good alignment. While I was doing balance exercises, the lack of core was preventing the balance exercises from working. It wasn't until after I applied the breathing techniques and my core began healing that I could begin seeing how crucial proprioception was to my daily living. I was once again able to make micro-adjustments.

With this encouraging news, I approached Olivia about trying balance exercises again. In 2023, Olivia assigned balance exercises beginning with me balancing on the floor.

BALANCE REHABILITATION EXERCISES

Notes: These exercises could be done sitting on an exercise ball, standing on the ground, or standing on a balance disc. Either the tactile side or the smooth side of the balance disc can be used. The advantage of the tactile side is it enhances balance control.[3] For this reason, it is suggested to perform all exercises barefoot.

Eyes Opened

Execution: Stand on the tactile side of a balance disc. Imagine a string pulling the head toward the ceiling to stand tall. Slightly tuck the chin. Inhale, verifying the back, sides, and chest are all moving with breath. Exhale, beginning from the abdomen. To assist with balance, squeeze the glutes and engage the core. Balance on the disc with the eyes open, for as long as possible.

Eyes Closed

Notes: A person can begin on the floor balancing with the eyes closed or use a balance disc.

Execution: Stand on the tactile side of a balance disc. Imagine a string pulling the head toward the ceiling to stand tall. Slightly tuck the chin. Inhale, verifying the back, sides, and chest are all moving with breath. Exhale, beginning from the abdomen. To assist with balance, squeeze the glutes and engage the core. Balance on the disc with the eyes closed, for as long as possible.

Turn Head

Notes: A person can begin on the floor balancing with the eyes closed or use a balance disc.

Execution: Stand on the tactile side of a balance disc. Imagine a string pulling the head toward the ceiling to stand tall. Slightly tuck the chin. Inhale, verifying the back, sides, and chest are all moving with breath. Exhale, beginning from the abdomen. To assist with balance, squeeze the glutes and engage the core. Maintain balance on the disc while turning the head slowly from side to side.

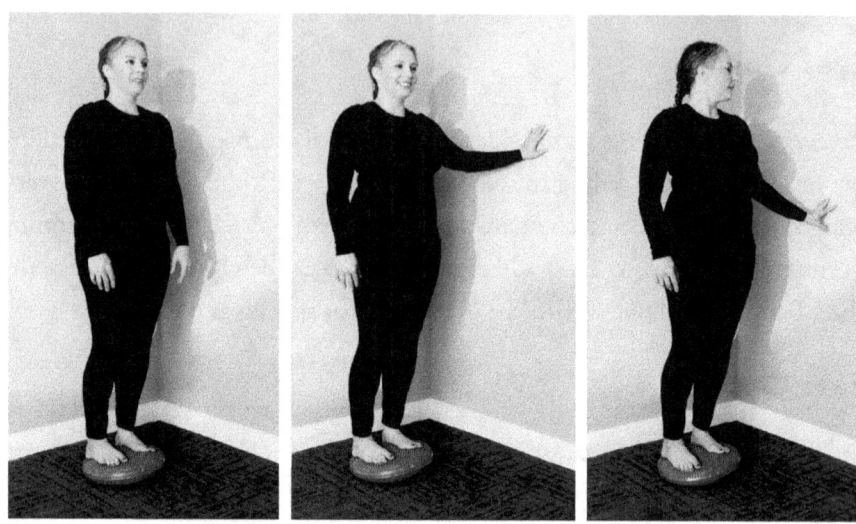

Figure 52. (*Left to right*) The model balances on the balance disk with eyes opened, eyes closed, and while turning the head.

Lift Leg

Notes: I was first asked to do this exercise in 2018. It seemed I was doing really great. At this time, I was only asked to do it standing on the floor. In 2019, I was asked to do it on a balance disc. However, I was in pain. I took a break for recovery for my core muscles. In 2023, I tried this pose on the balance disc again. Now, I know how many weakened muscles I had. When I began being required to use the correct muscles to balance, I had a much different result. I explained some issues I was having to Olivia in late 2023. She made me transition to the floor. Today, I can do this exercise without pain.

BALANCE REHABILITATION

Execution: Stand on the tactile side of a balance disc. Imagine a string pulling the head toward the ceiling to stand tall. Slightly tuck the chin. Inhale, verifying the back, sides, and chest are all moving with breath. Exhale, beginning from the abdomen. To assist with balance, squeeze the glute of the standing leg. Lift one leg. Hold and maintain balance. Lower. Repeat for the other leg.

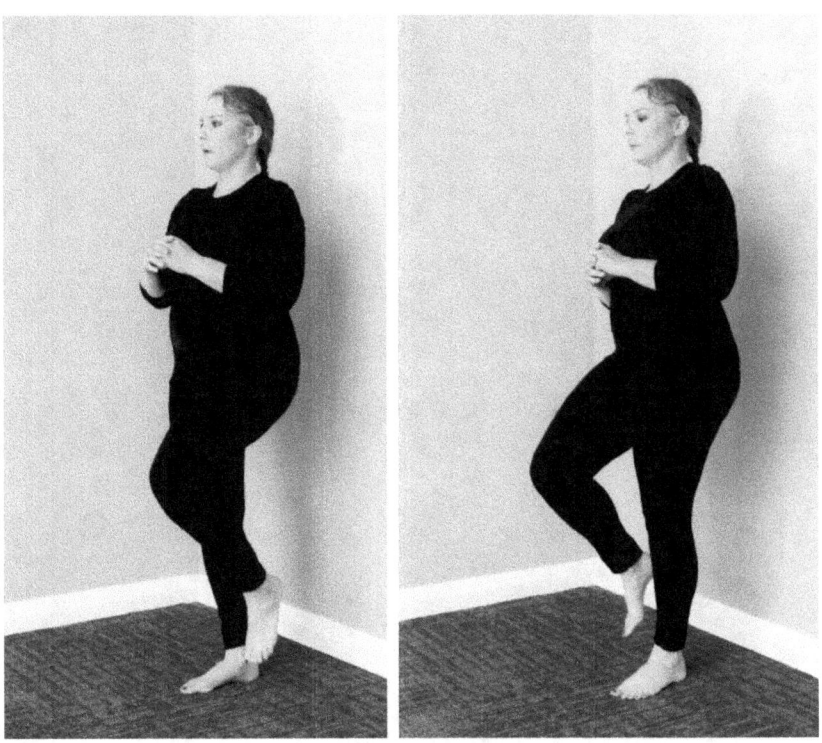

Figure 53. Lift leg.

26.
RUNNING REHABILITATION

In 2022, Olivia had me begin working toward one minute of running. I started with just a few seconds, such as 10 seconds of running at a time. I started running at 10 seconds with extended walk breaks of several minutes. It took a few weeks to work up to one minute of running. By late 2022, I was able to run 2-3 minutes. Then I signed up for my first 5k in the spring with the goal of running the whole race.

I focused on elbow planks and incline push-ups. I also began doing more leg and foot work as I noticed foot stiffness and began to develop Achilles issues. This introduced more rehabilitation. However, I was improving. I developed my three-month running plan. It involved exercise DVDs, yoga, and Essentrics.*

To be honest, it was really hard sticking to routine when working at Kohl's. Kohl's was so labor intensive that I was exhausted when I came home. I had little energy to do anything. When I started my new job, I had more energy and started to follow my plan. I was doing okay with running. When I had large increases in running times, I would feel the toll on my body. I thought this was a good sign.

Then, I ran my first mile. I focused on breathing, and I focused on using my core. I focused on maintaining good running form. I even maintained my desired pace. I had found a good pace. I was really happy and celebrated with each footfall as I looked at my Garmin and inched closer to the completion of my first mile after the tractor-trailer accident. Then, I reached my final footfall of that mile and started my cool down.

PAIN WITH POISE

Running Diary

February

Day	Distance	Description
8	3.5 miles	1 min run/3 min walk for 3.5 miles
11	2 miles	3 min run/3 min walk for 2 miles
15	3.5 miles	1 min run/3 min walk for 3.5 miles
18	2 miles	5 min run/3 min walk for 2 miles
22	3.5 miles	1 min run/3 min walk for 3.5 miles
25	2 miles	5 min run/3 min walk for 2 miles
29	3 miles	1 mile run/3 min walk for 3 miles

March

Day	Distance	Description
1	---	1 min run/3-4 min walk
4	---	5 min run/3 min walk/5 min run
8	1 mile	1 mile run
13	1 mile	1 mile run
16	---	0.5 mile run/0.25 mile walk/0.5 mile run
22	---	3.5 min walk/2 min run/2 min walk
25	1.5 miles	1.5 mile run
29	1 mile	1 mile run

Figure 54. My running diary from February to March when I trained for my first 5k after the tractor-trailer accident. The days I do not have a distance listed are the days I ran using my phone and didn't record a distance.

That was when I became alarmed. I began walking like a drunk. I wasn't dizzy. I wasn't light-headed. I didn't feel dehydrated. I took my left foot and placed it down and it stepped far to the left and I swung left. I took my right foot and placed it down and I stepped far to the right. So, I walked, like I was drunk down the sidewalk. The only thing I knew to do was try and fix my core. It wasn't ITBS. As I walked, I felt my thoracic spasm. While my thoracic spasm had improved over time, it hadn't vanished. Like a rubber band, I felt the pressure around my upper back, across my shoulder blades, and my chest.

I had spent years with a locked-up rib cage, spasms in my rib cage, and trying to undo the fascia. How do you fix this region? The other portions of my rib cage I had shoved my fingers into and all around the spaces of the ribs. I had a section I was certain would need more work. I contacted my chiropractor and got out my lacrosse ball and started focusing on my back. We needed a plan. I was assigned more breathing exercises and stretches by Olivia. (See breathing technique 3.)

I began a detox suggested by Dr. Craner. By the time I started Phase 2 of the detox, I had begun to notice a huge difference in energy levels. I was also beginning to notice a huge change in the strength of my core. Even with this, my legs were giving me huge problems. I was spending hours at home stretching with yoga, Essentrics˚, cupping, and using my massage gun and lacrosse ball.

Unfortunately, training didn't go as planned. I couldn't handle the mileage increases. My body was not healed enough for the mileage. I had to watch my pace to keep my heart rate under an acceptable pace. I mean, I had to run extremely slow. I had to majorly adjust my training schedule. I was thankful I had so much running experience from the past. I felt confident that with my adjustments I would be ready for race day and could still pull out a 5k.

My alarm went off at 5:15 a.m. on April 29, 2023. Race day was finally here. I got out of bed, prepped for the race, and left to pick up my race packet. I had a second where I was tired of the foot pain and said to myself, *Maybe I will never run again*. But, I got rid of that thought and prepared for race day. It turned out to be a drizzly day. It was the 20th Anniversary of the OhioHealth Capital City Half Marathon, and they were introducing the Columbus Promise 5k this year. Soon, we were off.

PAIN WITH POISE

I had started to develop a painful catch in an ankle in my last few weeks of runs. It didn't matter which ankle. It was just one of them. Within 10 feet of the starting line, my right ankle caught and sent a sharp pain. This time, I almost fell. I could just envision being *that* person who topples at the start line. I fought with all my might to stay upright. I was so weak that if I had gone down, the race would have been over. I almost didn't recover.

Running Diary

April

Day	Distance	Description
1	2 miles	2 mile run
5	1 miles	1 mile walk
8	2.25 miles	2.25 mile run
12	---	10 min run/10 min walk (x2)
15	2.5 miles	2.5 min run
27	0.5 miles	0.5 mile run
29	3.1 miles	3.1 mile run

Figure 55. My running diary from April when I trained for my first 5k after the tractor-trailer accident. The days I do not have a distance listed are the days I ran using my phone and didn't record a distance.

Somehow, I found a might in me to stay up, and I progressed along the course. This day, I was really concerned as my pace was far too fast. I had trained for a pace of 15:00 minute per mile (MM) and I was in the 12s. I struggled with my pace the whole race. I never got it down to my needed pace. As I expected, my lower core and lower body strength gave

RUNNING REHABILITATION

out. I shuffled along. Somehow, I pushed through. I barely made it. I felt like death when I crossed the finish line. Runners do things they should not. However, I finished my race that day. I felt like it, too.

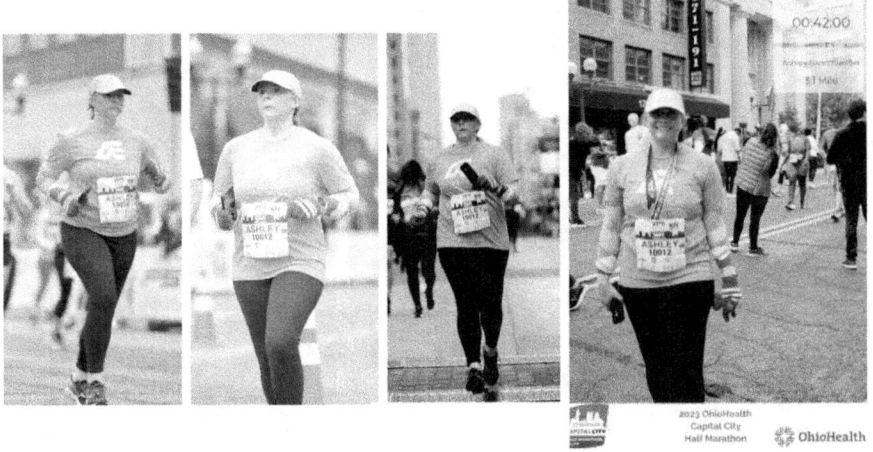

Figure 56. OhioHealth Columbus Promise 5k[1]

27.
RESOURCES & THE SCIENCE OF THE ACCIDENT

For starters, I considered the kinetic energy of the accident. To simplify the physics and because I did not have all the variables, such as distance vehicles traveled, I chose to consider the impacting vehicle's energy. Both mass and velocity would affect the initial kinetic energy of a motor vehicle accident. Initial kinetic energy, KE, is half of the mass, m, of the moving vehicle times its velocity, v, squared.

$$KE = 1/2mv^2 \quad (i)$$

As shown in Table I, if the mass of an 18-wheeler was 40 tons and the velocity was 50 mph, then the kinetic energy at impact would be 9.0647 MN. In comparison, a tractor-trailer of the same mass but traveling at 15 mph would have a kinetic energy of 0.81592 MN while a tractor-trailer moving at 65 mph would have a kinetic energy of 15.320 MN. A car, with a mass of 2 tons, would have a kinetic energy of 0.453 MN at 50 mph and 0.0408 MN at 15 mph, respectively. In Table I, the scenario that most closely resembles my accident is shaded in gray.

	Tractor-trailer			Car		
Mass of Vehicle (ton)	40	40	40	2	2	2
Mass of Vehicle (kg)	36,287	36,287	36,287	1,814.4	1,814.4	1,814.4
Velocity of Vehicle (mph)	65.0	50.0	15.0	65.0	50.0	15.0
Velocity of Vehicle (m/s)	29.058	22.352	6.706	29.058	22.352	6.706
Kinetic Energy (MN)	15.320	9.0647	0.81592	0.76601	0.45325	0.040797

Table I. Kinetic energies of vehicles traveling at 65, 50 and 15 mph[1]

After reviewing the increases in kinetic energy, there was clearly a significant increase between the initial increase in mass between the car and semi-trailer truck. Therefore, for a person in a vehicle hit by a semi-truck at any velocity, it greatly increased their rate of severe injury. The kinetic energy of a fully loaded (40 ton) tractor-trailer traveling at 15 mph has similar kinetic energy of a car (2 ton) traveling at 65 mph. The impact of a much more massive vehicle, such as a tractor-trailer, on a human body is significant even at very low velocities.

If the mass was held constant while the velocity was increased, the kinetic energy would increase exponentially. In fact, the velocity affects the kinetic energy more than the mass of the moving vehicle because the velocity increases exponentially, unlike the mass. Therefore, even tiny increases in velocity could result in more severe injuries, as it has a significant effect on the magnitude of the kinetic energy.[2] To show this change, a velocity squared differential and a mass times velocity squared differential (MTVSD) was evaluated in Table II. The velocity squared differential, VSD, is the difference of the velocity squared of vehicle A, v^2_A, from the velocity squared of vehicle B, v^2_B.

$$VSD = v^2_B - v^2_A \quad (ii)$$

Then, the mass times velocity squared differential, MTVSD, is the mass, m, times the velocity squared differential, VSD. The MTVSD shows a change in velocity from 15 mph to 65 mph has a significant change for the car and an exorbitant change for the semi-trailer truck. The enormous change in magnitude, observed by changing the 18-wheeler's velocity, is untouchable—the car's MTVSD cannot come close at any VSD. Even a much smaller change in the semi-trailer truck's velocity, such as from 50 to 65 mph, results in a magnitude increase that is greater than any of the car's MTVSD, as shown in Table II. These calculations support the conclusion that vehicles of similar mass can incur more human damage by traveling at much higher rates of velocities, as this significantly increases the energy the human body must absorb.

While velocity would affect the kinetic energy more than the vehicle mass, the mass still mattered. A highly massive vehicle has much more kinetic energy than a less massive vehicle at any velocity. However, the greater the initial mass of the vehicle, the more the MTVSD will be affected. Once a high rate of velocity has been reached, mass is even more dangerous. For this reason, the mass of the vehicle is extremely important and must be taken into consideration even when treating a patient. Mass is the source that catapults the velocity to its most dangerous level. This is the evolution of the high impact injury.

	Tractor-trailer			Car		
	A	B	C	D	E	F
Kinetic Energy (MN)	15.320	9.0647	0.81592	0.76601	0.45325	0.040797
Mass of Vehicle (kg)	36,287	36,287	36,287	1,814.4	1,814.4	1,814.4
Velocity of Vehicle (mph)	65.0	50.0	15.0	65.0	50.0	15.0
Velocity of Vehicle (m/s)	29.058	22.352	6.706	29.058	22.352	6.706
Velocity Squared Differential	344.75	454.64	—	344.75	454.64	—
Mass x Differential	12,510,000	16,497,000	—	625,510	824,900	—

Table II. Product of Mass and Velocity Squared Differential

So far, a simplistic energetic perspective has been presented. In real life, no accident is simple. For example, my vehicle was turning in the opposite direction of the semi-trailer truck's direction when it impacted my car. It was also an oblique crash[3] as the angle at impact was less than 90⁰. This actually increased the kinetic energy of the accident as the two vehicles at impact were traveling toward each other at velocity. If this had been a head-on collision, the kinetic energy would have been twice a rear impact.[4]

I believe I gassed my car at the time of impact. This is because my last driving thought was of transferring my foot from the brake to the gas pedal to accelerate into the turn. Therefore, I was actually increasing the speed of my car at impact. As I lost consciousness at that time, I don't know what my foot did. It could have stayed lodged on the gas pedal or it could have been forced off the gas pedal. If my foot stayed lodged on the gas pedal, this would've increased the friction between the two vehicles and my car tires and the road.

RESOURCES & THE SCIENCE OF THE ACCIDENT

What happened with all of this kinetic energy? It transformed into other forms, such as sound energy, heat energy, or deformation energy.[5] Signs of energy loss were anywhere deformations resulted upon impact.[6] Energy was also absorbed by the passengers in the vehicle. This also resulted in deformations of the human. There was no such thing as an energy shield in the accident. The human was part of the car at impact. The human energy form would absorb the energy upon collision while the remaining kinetic energy would transform into other energy forms.

To evaluate the energy my body absorbed, I visualized the accident as an energy field.[7] I decided to apply it to the accident scene to try and envision what happened to me. As I envisioned the accident scene as energy fields, I saw the semi-truck as energy. My car was energy. I was energy. The air was energy. Upon applying this energy visual, I no longer saw boundaries separating a human body from a car seat or from air, but now I could see energy transferring from one energy form to another with ease. And, a blast of energy was being absorbed by a human body.

Other factors that influenced how much energy my body absorbed were how much my car resisted being moved. The more my car resisted being moved, the more my body absorbed energy. The less my car resisted being moved, the less energy my body absorbed. When the tractor-trailer impacted my car, it transferred energy to my car, which then accelerated the vehicle. This process transferred some of the kinetic energy from the semi-trailer truck to my car. At the same time, there was resistance in the accident. My car did not want to move. This friction actually increased the energy my car absorbed because it did not easily move. The more time an object is in contact with the impacting object, the more damage will be sustained because more energy is absorbed. Time is an essential dimension.

Cars are designed to absorb the majority of the energy to protect the human. First, cars are made of steel alloys. Not all steel alloys are made the same. Steel alloy properties, such as strength and hardness, are dependent on the percentage of iron and other alloy elements used in the steel alloy with which the car is manufactured. Some steel alloys handle stress and deformation better than other steel alloys. For this reason, some cars are built better for accidents. This allows for cars to better absorb energy for passengers.

Because of Newton's law of motion, the force at impact moved my car in an opposite but equal direction. This means my body and organs accelerated with the vehicle in an equal and opposite direction. It was this unexpected burst of energy that caused damage to my car and body. The direction of the force affects the body and each component of the body differently.

THE NEURAL NETWORK

To put a grammatically correct sentence together stresses the brain. It is a cognitive exercise. We begin developing sentences as children. This is natural and develops a healthy neural network. When a person's brain is taxed from a concussion accumulated with pain and trauma, putting together a sentence is not the same. A neuron may be damaged. The neural network will malfunction. This will result in cognitive deficits. With the added stress, it will malfunction more. More neurons may be damaged.

Here's an example with the visual of a sidewalk full of runners…

To format a grammatically correct sentence, a healthy neural network transmits an electrical signal along the network. This signal relays the sentence and muscle synergy. In a dysfunctioning neural network, a storm (inflammation) blows into the neural network (sidewalk of runners). The wind blows debris and rain into the running group. The runners (electrical signal) can't see (confusion, pain!). The runners get disconnected (fear, confusion, pain!). The runners' pace changes depending on the obstacles and the direction of the wind. Some run faster (increased energy = pain!) and some run slower (decreased energy = pain!). The storm blows the runners off course (confusion, curse word).

The runners try to reunite (pain, increase energy!) with their bruised, (stretched axon) bleeding, and broken bones (broken axon). Persistent,

RESOURCES & THE SCIENCE OF THE ACCIDENT

they still struggle to arrive at their destination (cognitive exhaustion). In the meantime, some runners use their phones to call friends for help (the brain borrows from other areas of the brain). The running group finally reaches their destination and relays their message. But, the sentence is jumbled and the muscles may not work correctly. The speaker is exhausted and crippled in pain.

ACKNOWLEDGMENTS

I relied on a great team of medical experts for the writing of this book. I am extremely grateful for the expertise of Dr. Craner, Dr. Murphy, Olivia, and James Fryer. Dr. Craner offered her anatomical expertise and provided editorial contributions. Dr. Murphy introduced me to how he practices chiropractic and provided valuable information to my questions. Olivia reviewed the exercises to include for this book. James Fryer spent an early morning over coffee for an interview providing additional perspectives and clarification on breathing functionality. A special thank you to the Merrithew® team and Essentrics® team for providing editorial support.

I'm so thankful Natalie Sexton agreed to do my photos and Murphy Chiropractic & Performance Center opened up their practice on a Saturday morning for us. Natalie met me in the early morning, dealt with the blazing morning sun, and waited patiently on me to figure out how to do an exercise photo. We rearranged MCPC, used all the rooms, and put it back together. We even had to use the parking lot for photo props. Active Edge Chiropractic & Functional Medicine was also used as a photography location for a few last-minute pictures. Without the generosity of all, the exercise photos would never have materialized. Natalie can be contacted at www.nsextonphotography.com.

The custom artwork was created by Charis, an illustrator with six years of experience, and Tasnia Tarana, a graphic designer with over ten years of experience in medical and academic illustration. Their collaboration, creativity, and experience made my ideas a reality. I'm so thankful for them.

Thank you to my friends Gina and Randy. They brought me fun in the dark. Thank you to my running buddy forever, Carey. He inspired me to write this book. Without him, this book would never have happened. He always believed in me.

Thank you to the many people all over the world who have listened to me.

Lastly, thank you to my family. I have too many things to add here, so I will sum it up with I was blessed to have more time with you.

BIBLIOGRAPHY

Active Edge Chiropractic & Functional Medicine. "Dry Needling Therapy Columbus Ohio - Active Edge Chiropractic," October 6, 2020, accessed on October 24, 2023. https://columbuschiropractors.com/dry-needling-care-ohio/.

Astuti, Cahyaning Puji, Melyana Nurul Widyawati, and Suryono Suryono. "Application Model of Pranic Healing Therapy for Emotional Stress Using Accurate Bio-Well GDV Camera." *E3S Web of Conferences* 125 (January 1, 2019): 05005. https://doi.org/10.1051/e3sconf/201912505005. (CC BY 4.0 Deed | Attribution 4.0 International | Creative Commons).

Breit, Sigrid, Aleksandra Kupferberg, Gerhard Rogler, and Gregor Hasler. "Vagus Nerve as Modulator of the Brain–Gut Axis in Psychiatric and Inflammatory Disorders." *Frontiers in Psychiatry* 9 (March 13, 2018). https://doi.org/10.3389/fpsyt.2018.00044. (CC BY 4.0 Deed | Attribution 4.0 International | Creative Commons).

Chen, Yanjiao, Cai-Tao Chen, Jiayuan Liu, Gabriel Shimizu Bassi, and Yongqing Yang. "What Is the Appropriate Acupuncture Treatment Schedule for Chronic Pain? Review and Analysis of Randomized Controlled Trials." *Evidence-Based Complementary and Alternative Medicine* 2019 (June 18, 2019): 1–10. https://doi.org/10.1155/2019/5281039. (CC BY 4.0 Deed | Attribution 4.0 International | Creative Commons).

Chi, Hongpeng, and Bing Gong. "Analysis of Energy Conversion Law in Vehicle Collision Accident." *Journal of Physics: Conference Series* 1486, no. 7 (April 1, 2020): 072014. https://doi.org/10.1088/1742-6596/1486/7/072014. (CC BY 3.0 Deed | Attribution 3.0 Unported | Creative Commons).

Chou, Ping-Song, Yu-Chi Huang, and Sebastian Yu. "Mechanisms of Epigenetic Inheritance in Post-Traumatic Stress Disorder." *Life* 14, no. 1 (January 8, 2024): 98. https://doi.org/10.3390/life14010098. (CC BY 4.0 Deed | Attribution 4.0 International | Creative Commons).

De Cássia Vieira, Rita, Wellingson Silva Paiva, Daniel Oliveira, Manoel Jacobsen Teixeira, Almir Ferreira De Andrade, and Regina Márcia Cardoso De Sousa. "Diffuse Axonal Injury: Epidemiology, Outcome and Associated Risk Factors." *Frontiers in Neurology* 7 (October 20, 2016). https://doi.org/10.3389/fneur.2016.00178. (CC BY 4.0 Deed | Attribution 4.0 International | Creative Commons).

DDP Yoga. "Never, ever give up. Arthur's inspirational transformation!" YouTube video, 4:54, April 30, 2012, https://www.youtube.com/watch?v=qX9FSZJu448. Used by permission.

Derrick Matthew Buchanan, Tomas Ros, and Richard Nahas, "Elevated and Slowed EEG Oscillations in Patients With Post-Concussive Syndrome and Chronic Pain Following a Motor Vehicle Collision," *Brain Sciences* 11, no. 5 (April 24, 2021): 537, https://doi.org/10.3390/brainsci11050537. (CC BY 4.0 Deed | Attribution 4.0 International | Creative Commons).

Downey, Adrian. "Split-Brain Syndrome and Extended Perceptual Consciousness." *Phenomenology and the Cognitive Sciences* 17, no. 4 (November 25, 2017): 787–811. https://doi.org/10.1007/s11097-017-9550-y. (CC BY 4.0 Deed | Attribution 4.0 International | Creative Commons).

BIBLIOGRAPHY

Essentrics®. "Build Your Core with Breathing - Essentrics®." Essentrics®, October 11, 2023, accessed on October 18, 2023. https://essentrics.com/build-your-core-with-breathing/. Used by permission.

Essentrics®. "Give Your Lungs a Chance: 3 Ways to Breathe Better - Essentrics®." Essentrics®, October 5, 2022, accessed on October 24, 2023. https://essentrics.com/3-ways-to-breathe-better-strong-lungs/. Used by permission.

Essentrics®. "The Science - Essentrics," September 6, 2022. https://essentrics.com/the-science/. Retrieved on 2023, October 22. Used by permission.

Essentrics®. "What Is Essentrics® - Essentrics®," (n.d.), accessed on October 24, 2023. https://essentrics.com/what-is-essentrics/. Used by permission.

Firouzjah, Morteza Homayounnia, Ebrahim Mohammad Ali Nasab Firouzjah, and Zahra Ebrahimi. "The Effect of a Course of Selected Corrective Exercises on Posture, Scapula-Humeral Rhythm and Performance of Adolescent Volleyball Players with Upper Cross Syndrome." *BMC Musculoskeletal Disorders* 24, no. 1 (June 14, 2023). https://doi.org/10.1186/s12891-023-06592-7. (CC BY 4.0 Deed | Attribution 4.0 International | Creative Commons).

Georgiev, Georgi Zdravkov. "Impact Force Calculator - Calculate the Impact Force in a Collision." www.gigacalculator.com, n.d. https://www.gigacalculator.com/calculators/impact-force-calculator.php.

Hometown Stations. "One Transported to Hospital after Semi vs Car Crash," May 15, 2018. Accessed June 6, 2021. https://www.hometownstations.com/news/one-transported-to-hospital-after-semi-vs-car-crash/article_c9ce5381-dc79-5f9b-9f44-bd8a1bd077e8.html. Used by permission.

Huang, Jianpeng, Zhan-Mou Liang, Qi-Wen Zou, Jianming Zhan, Wenting Li, Sheng Li, Kai Li, Wen Fu, and Jianhua Liu. "Electroacupuncture on Hemifacial Spasm and Temporomandibular Joint Pain Co-Morbidity: A Case Report." *Frontiers in Neurology* 13 (June 28, 2022). https://doi.org/10.3389/fneur.2022.931412. (CC BY 4.0 Deed | Attribution 4.0 International | Creative Commons).

"HUB - Enmotive Race Day Results and Photos - Raceday@enmotive," April 27, 2023, https://raceday.enmotive.com/#/events/2023-ohio-health-capital-city-half-marathon/registrants/f0a93203-34ea-4676-9449-e15dde50d9e1. Used by permission.

Kenzie, Erin S., Elle L. Parks, Erin D. Bigler, Miranda M. Lim, J. C. Chesnutt, and Wayne W. Wakeland. "Concussion as a Multi-Scale Complex System: An Interdisciplinary Synthesis of Current Knowledge." *Frontiers in Neurology* 8 (September 28, 2017). https://doi.org/10.3389/fneur.2017.00513. (CC BY 4.0 Deed | Attribution 4.0 International | Creative Commons).

Khera, Tanvi, and Valluvan Rangasamy. "Cognition and Pain: A Review." *Frontiers in Psychology* 12 (May 21, 2021). https://doi.org/10.3389/fpsyg.2021.673962. (CC BY 4.0 Deed | Attribution 4.0 International | Creative Commons).

Khorasani-Zavareh, Davoud, Maryam Bigdeli, Soheil Saadat, and Reza Mohammadi. "Kinetic Energy Management in Road Traffic Injury Prevention: A Call for Action." *Journal of Injury and Violence Research*, July 1, 2014. https://jivresearch.org/jivr/index.php/jivr/article/view/458. (CC BY 3.0 Deed | Attribution 3.0 Unported | Creative Commons).

BIBLIOGRAPHY

Khouri, Charles, Matthieu Roustit, and Jean-Luc Cracowski. "Impact of Global Warming on Raynaud's Phenomenon: A Modelling Study." *F1000Research* 9 (July 30, 2020): 829. https://doi.org/10.12688/f1000research.24939.1. (CC BY 4.0 Deed | Attribution 4.0 International | Creative Commons).

Klein, Willis B., Suzanne Wood, and Jennifer Bartz. 2023. "You Think I'm Insane: An Integrative Review and Novel Theoretical Framework for Studying the Phenomenon of Gaslighting." PsyArXiv. August 23. https://doi.org/10.31234/osf.io/gs5mp. (CC BY 4.0 Deed | Attribution 4.0 International | Creative Commons).

Komariah, Maria, Kusman Ibrahim, Tuti Pahria, Laili Rahayuwati, and Irman Somantri. "Effect of Mindfulness Breathing Meditation on Depression, Anxiety, and Stress: A Randomized Controlled Trial among University Students." *Healthcare* 11, no. 1 (December 22, 2022): 26. https://doi.org/10.3390/healthcare11010026. (CC BY 4.0 Deed | Attribution 4.0 International | Creative Commons).

Lacal, Irene, Ventura, Rossella. "Epigenetic Inheritance: Concepts, Mechanisms and Perspectives." *Frontiers in Molecular Neuroscience* 11 (September 28, 2018). https://doi.org/10.3389/fnmol.2018.00292. (CC BY 4.0 Deed | Attribution 4.0 International | Creative Commons).

Li, Weihui, and Andrew Ahn. "Subcutaneous Fascial Bands—A Qualitative and Morphometric Analysis." *PLOS ONE* 6, no. 9 (September 8, 2011): e23987. https://doi.org/10.1371/journal.pone.0023987. (CC BY 4.0 Deed | Attribution 4.0 International | Creative Commons).

Lincoln, Abraham, Pres. U.S. Gettysburg address delivered at Gettysburg Pa. Nov. 19th, .n. p. n. d. PDF. https://www.loc.gov/item/rbpe.24404500/.

Merrithew˚. "The STOTT PILATES˚ Basic Principles: Breathing," n.d., accessed on October 18, 2023, https://www.merrithew.com/stott-pilates/warmup/en/principles/breathing#:~:text=Focus%20on%20sending%20breath%20into,cage%20and%20encouraging%20full%20expansion. Used by permission.

Meyer, Stephen M., Heidi Stöckl, Cecilia Vorfeld, Kaloyan Kamenov, and ClaudíA Garcia-Moreno. "A Scoping Review of Measurement of Violence Against Women and Disability." *PLOS ONE* 17, no. 1 (January 31, 2022): e0263020. https://doi.org/10.1371/journal.pone.0263020. (CC BY 4.0 Deed | Attribution 4.0 International | Creative Commons).

Nia, Arastoo, Domenik Popp, Cornelia Diendorfer, Sebastian Apprich, Alexandru Munteanu, Stefan Hajdu, and Harald Widhalm. "Impact of Lockdown during the COVID-19 Pandemic on Number of Patients and Patterns of Injuries at a Level I Trauma Center." *Wiener Klinische Wochenschrift* 133, no. 7–8 (March 3, 2021): 336–43. https://doi.org/10.1007/s00508-021-01824-z. (CC BY 4.0 Deed | Attribution 4.0 International | Creative Commons).

Pascal, Blaise, *The Thoughts of Blaise Pascal: translated from the text of M. Auguste Molinier* trans. by C. Kegan Paul, Urbana, Illinois: The Project Gutenberg, 2014. First published 1885 by Kegan Paul, Trench & Co. Retrieved February 21, 2016, from https://www.https://www.gutenberg.org/ebooks/46921.

Prentkovskis, Olegas, Edgar Sokolovskij, and Vilius Bartulis. "Investigating Traffic Accidents: A Collision of two motor vehicles." *Transport* 25, no. 2 (June 30, 2010): 105–15. https://doi.org/10.3846/transport.2010.14. (CC BY 4.0 Deed | Attribution 4.0 International | Creative Commons).

BIBLIOGRAPHY

Shah, Riddhi. Merrithew®. "What Is a Pilates Reformer?," Merrithew® Blog, August 22, 2023, accessed on October 6, 2023. https://www.merrithew.com/blog/post/2023-08-22/what-is-a-pilates-reformer. Used by permission.

Shelley, Mary. "Frankenstein, or the Modern Prometheus." In *Amsterdam University Press eBooks*, 2018. https://doi.org/10.1515/9781942401223-029.

Singh, Rajat Emanuel, Kamran Iqbal, Gannon White, and Tarun E. Hutchinson. "A Systematic Review on Muscle Synergies: From Building Blocks of Motor Behavior to a Neurorehabilitation Tool." *Applied Bionics and Biomechanics* 2018 (January 1, 2018): 1–15. https://doi.org/10.1155/2018/3615368. (CC BY 4.0 Deed | Attribution 4.0 International | Creative Commons).

Wang, Chunni, Shengli Guo, Ying Xu, Jun Ma, Jun Tang, Faris Alzahrani, and Aatef Hobiny. "Formation of Autapse Connected to Neuron and Its Biological Function." *Complexity* 2017 (January 1, 2017): 1–9. https://doi.org/10.1155/2017/5436737. (CC BY 4.0 Deed | Attribution 4.0 International | Creative Commons).

Wang, Qi, and Haitao Fu. "Relationship between Proprioception and Balance Control among Chinese Senior Older Adults." *Frontiers in Physiology* 13 (December 15, 2022). https://doi.org/10.3389/fphys.2022.1078087. (CC BY 4.0 Deed | Attribution 4.0 International | Creative Commons).

Yang, Changju, Yi Du, Jianbin Wu, Jun Wang, Ping Luan, Qin-Lao Yang, and Lin Yuan. "Fascia and Primo Vascular System." *Evidence-Based Complementary and Alternative Medicine* 2015 (January 1, 2015): 1–6. https://doi.org/10.1155/2015/303769. (CC BY 3.0 Deed | Attribution 3.0 Unported | Creative Commons).

Yi, Meisheng, Jing Li, Gang Liu, Zilin Ou, Yanmei Liu, Jing Li, Zhong Chen, et al. "Mental Health and Quality of Life in Patients with Craniofacial Movement Disorders: A Cross-Sectional Study." *Frontiers in Neurology* 13 (September 21, 2022). https://doi.org/10.3389/fneur.2022.938632. (CC BY 4.0 Deed | Attribution 4.0 International | Creative Commons).

Zhao, Yixuan, Ze Chen, Longfei Li, Xipeng Wu, and Wei Li. "Changes in Proprioception at Different Time Points Following Anterior Cruciate Ligament Injury or Reconstruction." *Journal of Orthopaedic Surgery and Research* 18, no. 1 (July 31, 2023). https://doi.org/10.1186/s13018-023-04044-5. (CC BY 4.0 Deed | Attribution 4.0 International | Creative Commons).

Zhou, Jingtian, Zhuzhu Zhang, May Wu, Hanqing Liu, Yan Pang, A. Bartlett, Zihao Peng, et al. "Brain-wide Correspondence of Neuronal Epigenomics and Distant Projections." *Nature* 624, no. 7991 (December 13, 2023): 355–65. https://doi.org/10.1038/s41586-023-06823-w. (CC BY 4.0 Deed | Attribution 4.0 International | Creative Commons).

ENDNOTES

PREFACE

1. Blaise Pascal, *The Thoughts of Blaise Pascal: translated. from the text of M. Auguste Molinier,* trans. by C. Kegan Paul, (1885, reis., The Project Gutenberg, 2014).

2. Shelley, Mary. "Frankenstein, or the Modern Prometheus." In *Amsterdam University Press eBooks*, 2018, 179-82.

CHAPTER ONE

1. Daniela Ismerio, email communication to Ashley Swartzwelder, October 29, 2023.

2. Note. 2018. [Photograph]. © Copyright 2024 https://www.hometownstations.com/news/one-transported-to-hospital-after-semi-vs-car-crash/article_c9ce5381-dc79-5f9b-9f44-bd8a1bd077e8.html Retrieved June 6, 2021.

CHAPTER THREE

1. Essentrics®. (n.d.). Adapted from *The Science Behind Essentrics®.* https://essentrics.com/the-science/ (Copyright 2019 by The Esmonde Technique). Retrieved on 2023, October 22.

2. Yang, C., Du, Y., Wu, J., Wang, J., Luan, P., Yang, Q., & Yuan, L.

(2015). New developments in primo vascular system: imaging and functions with regard to acupuncture. *Evidence-Based Complementary and Alternative Medicine,* 2015 Article 303769. http://dx.doi.org/10.1155/2015/303769 (http://creativecommons.org/licenses/by-sa/3.0/).; Craner, personal communication, August 2021.

3. The average force was calculated assuming the 36,287 kg tractor-trailer was traveling 22.352 m/s resulting in my vehicle being moved 1 m during a 1 second impact duration using an Impact Force Calculator (Gigacalculator. (n.d.) *Impact Force Calculator.*)

4. Wang, C., Guo, S., Xu, Y., Ma, J. (2017). Formation of autapse connected to neuron and its biological function. *Complexity,* 2017, Article 5436737. https://doi.org/10.1155/2017/5436737.

5. I developed Raynaud's phenomenon as a teenager in my fingers. This phenomena can occur under stressful situations or when exposed to certain weather conditions. The blood vessels in the fingers or toes overreact and go white and numb. Essentially, the vessels spasm (Khouri, Charles, Roustit, Matthieu, Cracowski, Jean-Luc. (2020). Impact of global warming on Raynaud's phenomenon: a modeling study [version 1; peer review: 2 approved]. *F1000Research* 2020, 9:829. https://doi.org/10.12688/f1000research.24939.1.

6. Khera, T., & Rangasamy, V. (2021). Cognition and pain: a review. *Frontiers in psychology,* 12, Article 673962. https://doi.org/10.3389/fpsyg.2021.673962

7. Lincoln, Abraham, Pres. U. S. Gettysburg address delivered at Gettysburg Pa. Nov. 19th.

8. Derrick Matthew Buchanan, Tomas Ros, and Richard Nahas, "Elevated and Slowed EEG Oscillations in Patients With Post-Concussive Syndrome and Chronic Pain Following a Motor Vehicle Collision," *Brain Sciences* 11, no. 5 (April 24, 2021): 537, https://doi.org/10.3390/brainsci11050537.

ENDNOTES

9. Erin S. Kenzie et al., "Concussion as a Multi-Scale Complex System: An Interdisciplinary Synthesis of Current Knowledge," *Frontiers in Neurology* 8 (September 28, 2017), https://doi.org/10.3389/fneur.2017.00513.

10. ibid.

11. Rita De Cássia Vieira et al., "Diffuse Axonal Injury: Epidemiology, Outcome and Associated Risk Factors," *Frontiers in Neurology* 7 (October 20, 2016), https://doi.org/10.3389/fneur.2016.00178.

12. Wang et al., "Formation of Autapse Connected to Neuron and Its Biological Function."

13. ibid.

CHAPTER FIVE

1. Matt. 27:46 (New King James Version)

2. Downey, A. (2018). Split-brain syndrome and extended perceptual consciousness. *Phenom. Cogn. Sci.* 17, 787–811. https://doi.org/10.1007/s11097-017-9550-y.

3. Matthew 27:46 (NKJV)

4. Job 10:1-22 (NKJV)

5. Exod. 32:19 (NKJV)

6. Exod. 34:29-33 (NKJV)

7. Luke 22:44 (NKJV)

CHAPTER SEVEN

1. Irene Lacal and Rossella Ventura, "Epigenetic Inheritance: Concepts, Mechanisms and Perspectives," *Frontiers in Molecular Neuroscience* 11 (September 28, 2018), https://doi.org/10.3389/fnmol.2018.00292; Ping-Song Chou, Yu-Chi Huang, and Sebastian Yu, "Mechanisms of Epigenetic Inheritance in Post-Traumatic Stress Disorder," *Life* 14, no. 1 (January 8, 2024): 98, https://doi.org/10.3390/life14010098.

CHAPTER NINE

1. Klein, Willis B., Suzanne Wood, and Jennifer Bartz. 2023. "You Think I'm Insane: An Integrative Review and Novel Theoretical Framework for Studying the Phenomenon of Gaslighting." PsyArXiv. August 23. https://doi.org/10.31234/osf.io/gs5mp.

2. Klein, "You Think I'm Insane: An Integrative Review and Novel Theoretical Framework for Studying the Phenomenon of Gaslighting," 8.

3. ibid.

4. This is the same neurological nurse who wrongfully accused me of having reactions to my medications, because they canceled the wrong person's appointment.

CHAPTER TWELVE

1. Warner, Anna. "Jesus Loves Me." *Church Hymnal*, 1951, p. 87.

ENDNOTES

CHAPTER THIRTEEN

1. Arastoo MD, Nia, Domenik Popp, MD, Cornelia Diendorfer, Sebastian Apprich, MD, Alexandru Munteanu, MBBS, Stefan Hajdu, MD, and Harald K. Widhalm, MD, PhD. "*Impact of lockdown during the COVID-19 pandemic on number of patients and patterns of injuries at a level I trauma center.*" Wien Klin Wochenschr 133 no. 7 (Mar. 2021): 336–343. https://doi: 10.1007/s00508-021-01824-z.

CHAPTER FOURTEEN

1. Li W, Ahn AC. (2011). Subcutaneous Fascial Bands—A Qualitative and Morphometric Analysis. PLoS ONE 6(9), Article e23987. https://doi.org/10.1371/journal.pone.0023987.

2. *Trademark or registered trademark of Merrithew International Inc., used under license.

3. Shah, Riddhi. (2023, August 22). What is a Pilates Reformer? Merrithew®. https://www.merrithew.com/blog/post/2023-08-22/what-is-a-pilates-reformer. Adapted by permission.

4. Jingtian Zhou et al., "Brain-wide Correspondence of Neuronal Epigenomics and Distant Projections," Nature 624, no. 7991 (December 13, 2023): 355–65, https://doi.org/10.1038/s41586-023-06823-w.

CHAPTER SIXTEEN

1. DDP Yoga. (2012, April 30). *Never, ever give up. Arthur's inspirational transformation!* [Video]. YouTube. https://www.youtube.com/watch?v=qX9FSZJu448. Used by permission.

PART 2 (OPENING QUOTE)

Dr. Leon Kass, email communication to Ashley Swartzwelder, October 30, 2023.

CHAPTER EIGHTEEN

1. Singh, R., Iqbal, K., White, G., Edgar, T. (2018). A systematic review on muscle synergies: from building blocks of motor behavior to a neurorehabilitation tool. *Applied Bionics and Biomechanics,* 2018, Article 3615368. https://doi.org/10.1155/2018/3615368.

2. Khera and Rangasamy, "Cognition and Pain: A Review."

3. Komariah, M.; Ibrahim, K.; Pahria, T.; Rahayuwati, L.;Somantri, I. (2023) Effect of Mindfulness Breathing Meditation on Depression, Anxiety, and Stress: A Randomized Controlled Trial among University Students. *Healthcare, 11*(26). doi.org/10.3390/healthcare11010026.

4. Breit, S., Kupferberg, A., Rogler, G., & Hasler, G. (2018). Vagus Nerve as Modulator of the Brain-Gut Axis in Psychiatric and Inflammatory Disorders. *Frontiers in psychiatry, 9*, 44. https://doi.org/10.3389/fpsyt.2018.00044.

5. Chen, Yan-Jiao, Chen, Cai-Tao, Liu, Jia-Yuan, Bassi, Gabriel Shimizu, & Yang, Yong-Qing. (2019). What Is the appropriate acupuncture treatment schedule for chronic pain? Review and analysis of randomized controlled trials. *Evidence-Based Complementary and Alternative Medicine.* 2019, Article 5281039. doi.org/10.1155/2019/5281039.

6. (2016). Dry Needling Columbus Ohio. Active Edge Chiropractic & Functional Medicine. https://columbuschiropractors.com/dry-needling-care-ohio/ Retrieved on November 26, 2023.

ENDNOTES

7. Chen et al., "What Is the Appropriate Acupuncture Treatment Schedule for Chronic Pain? Review and Analysis of Randomized Controlled Trials."

8. Dry Needling, Active Edge Chiropractic & Functional Medicine.

9. Dry Needling, Active Edge Chiropractic & Functional Medicine.

10. Astuti, Cahyaning Puji, Widyawati, Melyana Nurul, & Suryono, Suryono. (2019). Application Model of Pranic Healing Therapy for Emotional Stress Using Accurate Bio-Well GDV Camera. *E3S Web of Conferences*. 125(1):05005. https://doi.org/10.1051/e3sconf/201912505005.

CHAPTER NINTEEN

1. *Note.* PHASE 1 of POISE is establishing a patient's framework for breathing. PHASE 2 begins functional rehabilitation in tiny, incremental steps. During the exercise, the patient will practice visualization. After trying the exercise, the patient will report pain felt and trauma released. The patient's report will determine the patient's progression. PHASE2 proceeds in forward steps (odd numbered arrows) with positive feedback and backward steps (even numbered arrows) with negative feedback. As the rehabilitation proceeds and the patient continues long-term care with his medical team, rest (PHASE 3) may be required in varying amounts due to inflammation, burnout, or side effects from prescribed medications. Insert: Illustrated by Tasnia Tarana, *Breathing*, Fiverr, March 19, 2024.

2. *Note.* Illustrated by Charis, *Dysfunctional and Functional*, Fiverr, March 21, 2024.

CHAPTER TWENTY

1. Essentrics˚. 2020, April 6. Give your lungs a chance: 3 ways to breathe better. https://essentrics.com/3-ways-to-breathe-better-strong-lungs/. ; Merrithew˚. (n.d.) The STOTT PILATES®* Basic Principles: Breathing. https://

www.merrithew.com/stott-pilates/warmup/en/principles/breathing#:~:text=-Focus on sending breath into,cage and encouraging full expansion.

2. Merrithew®, "The STOTT PILATES® Basic Principles: Breathing."

3. Essentrics®, "Build Your Core with Breathing - Essentrics®."

4. Merrithew®, "STOTT PILATES® Basic Principles: Breathing."

5. Bushway, Kathi. Essentrics®. Build your core with breathing. https://essentrics.com/build-your-core-with-breathing/.

6. Merrithew®, "STOTT PILATES® Basic Principles: Breathing."

7. *Note.* Illustrated by Tasnia Tarana, *Breathing*, Fiverr, March 19, 2024.

CHAPTER TWENTY-ONE

1. Bushway, Essetnrics®, Core.

CHAPTER TWENTY-TWO

1. Craner.

2. Fu, Wen-bin, Jian-peng Huang, Kai Li, Sheng Li, Wen-ting Li, Zhan-mou Liang, and Jian-hua Liu. "Electroacupuncture on hemifacial spasm and temporomandibular joint pain co-morbidity: a case report." *Front. Neurology* no. 13 (June 2022): article: 931412. https://doi.org/10.3389/fneur.2022.931412.

3. Chen, Yicong, Chao Dang, Yaomin Guo, Jing Li, Jing Li, Gang Liu, and Yanmei Liu. "Mental health and quality of life in patients with craniofacial movement disorders: A cross-sectional study." *Front. Neurology* no. 13 (Sept. 2022): article 938632. https://doi.org/10.3389/fneur.2022.938632.

4. Adapted from Homayounnia Firouzjah, Morteza, Ebrahim Mohammad Ali Nasab Firouzjah, and Zahra Ebrahimi. "The effect of a course

of selected corrective exercises on posture, scapula-humeral rhythm and performance of adolescent volleyball players with upper cross syndrome." *BMC Musculoskeletal Disorders 489, no. 24* (June 2023). https://doi.org/10.1186/s12891-023-06592-7.

5. Wall short seated reach. Used by permission. Copyright © Postural Restoration Institute® 2023, www.posturalrestoration.com

CHAPTER TWENTY-FIVE

1. Wang, Q., Fu, H. (2022). Relationship between proprioception and balance control among Chinese senior older adults. *Front. Physiol.* 13:1078087. doi: 10.3389/fphys.2022.1078087.

2. Yixuan, Z., Ze, C. Long, L., Xipeng, W., & Wei, L. (2023). Changes in proprioception at different time points following anterior cruciate ligament injury or reconstruction. *Journal of Orthopedic Surgery and Research*, 18(547). https://doi.org/10.1186/s13018-023-04044-5.

3. Wang and Fu, "Relationship between Proprioception and Balance Control among Chinese Senior Older Adults."

CHAPTER TWENTY-SIX

1. *Note*. OhioHealth Columbus Promise 5k, [Photograph], From 2023 OhioHealth Capital City Half Marathon, 2023, Capital City Half Marathon. (https://raceday.enmotive.com/#/events/2023-ohiohealth-capital-city-half-marathon/registrants/f0a93203-34ea-4676-9449-e15d-de50d9e1). Used by permission.

CHAPTER TWENTY-SEVEN

1. *Note*. The kinetic energy, in megaNewton (MN), of two tractor-trailer and two car scenarios. The column shaded in gray is to guide the eye to

the variables the tractor-trailer was traveling during my motor vehicle accident.

2. Chi, H., Gong, B. (2020). Analysis of energy conversion law in vehicle collision accident. *J. Phys.: Conf. Ser.* 1486 072014. doi: 10.1088/1742-6596/1486/7/072014.; Khorasani-Zavareh D, Bigdeli M, Saadat S, Mohammadi R. (2015). Kinetic energy management in road traffic injury prevention: a call for action. J Inj Violence Res.(1):36-7. https://jivresearch.org/jivr/index.php/jivr/article/view/458.

3. Prentkovskis, O., Sokolovskij, E., & Bartulis, V. (2010). Investigating traffic accidents: a collision of two motor vehicles. Transport. 25(2):105–115. doi: 10.3846/transport.2010.14.

4. Chi and Gong, "Analysis of Energy Conversion Law in Vehicle Collision Accident."

5. ibid.

6. Prentkovskis, Sokolovskij, and Bartulis, "Investigating Traffic Accidents: A Collision of two motor vehicles."

7. Years prior, I had begun visualizing the world as an energy field, such as a room. Instead of walls, I imagined an energy field. Instead of a table, it was an energy field. Instead of a floor, I imagined it being energy. The point was energy was everywhere.

ABOUT THE AUTHOR

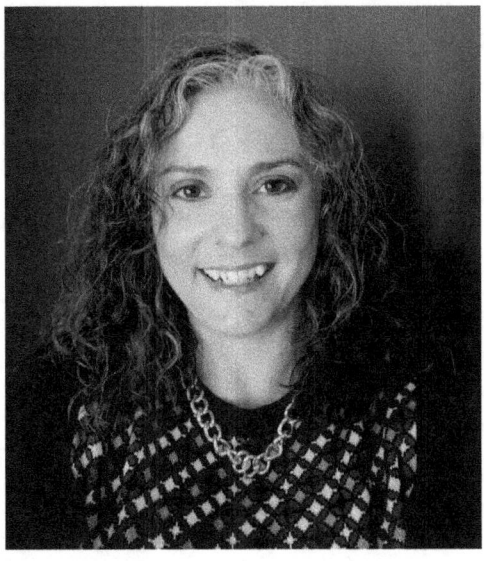

Ashley Swartzwelder specialized in water, atmospheric, and physical chemistry while earning her BS at Marshall University in Huntington, West Virginia, and her MS at The Ohio State University. During her 10-year tenure at Chemical Abstracts Service, she fully covered the STEM content developing an expertise in particle physics, nuclear engineering, analytical chemistry, geology, and health physics. She has also written chemistry content for Macmillan Learning.

In her spare time, she promotes awareness of domestic and international human rights violations. In 2017, she highlighted the brutality of North Korea's human rights violations with, "North Korean babies deserve to watch *Bambi* without being shot." She continues rehabbing to achieve her dreams of running the Marine Corps Marathon and to re-establish her career.

Learn more about Ashley at her website:
www.ashleyswartzwelder.com

www.ingramcontent.com/pod-product-compliance
Lightning Source LLC
Chambersburg PA
CBHW070047080526
44586CB00013B/944